Early Clinical Exposure
A Case Based Approach in
CLINICAL PHYSIOLOGY

Early Clinical Exposure
A Case Based Approach in
CLINICAL PHYSIOLOGY

As per the Competency-Based Medical Education Curriculum (NMC)

Manjinder Kaur
MBBS MD (Physiology) MAMS CMCL-FAIMER ACME Professional Certificate in Healthcare Management and Analytics (IIM Kozhikode)
Professor and Head
Department of Physiology
Additional Principal
Geetanjali Medical College and Hospital
Udaipur, Rajasthan, India

Co-Authors

Suman Sharma
MSc PhD (Medical Physiology) ACME
Professor
Department of Physiology
Geetanjali Medical College and Hospital
Udaipur, Rajasthan, India

Naren Kurmi
MBBS MD (Physiology)
Associate Professor
Department of Physiology
Government Medical College
Pali, Rajasthan, India

Sangita Chauhan
MBBS MD (Physiology)
Associate Professor
Department of Physiology
Geetanjali Medical College and Hospital
Udaipur, Rajasthan, India

JAYPEE

JAYPEE BROTHERS MEDICAL PUBLISHERS
The Health Sciences Publisher
New Delhi | London

Jaypee Brothers Medical Publishers (P) Ltd.

Headquarters
Jaypee Brothers Medical Publishers (P) Ltd
EMCA House
23/23-B, Ansari Road, Daryaganj
New Delhi - 110 002, India
Landline: +91-11-23272143, +91-11-23272703
+91-11-23282021, +91-11-23245672
Email: jaypee@jaypeebrothers.com

Corporate Office
Jaypee Brothers Medical Publishers (P) Ltd
4838/24, Ansari Road, Daryaganj
New Delhi 110 002, India
Phone: +91-11-43574357
Fax: +91-11-43574314
Email: jaypee@jaypeebrothers.com

Overseas Office
J.P. Medical Ltd
83 Victoria Street, London
SW1H 0HW (UK)
Phone: +44 20 3170 8910
Fax: +44 (0)20 3008 6180
Email: info@jpmedpub.com

Website: www.jaypeebrothers.com
Website: www.jaypeedigital.com

Inquiries for bulk sales may be solicited at: jaypee@jaypeebrothers.com

Early Clinical Exposure A Case Based Approach in Clinical Physiology

First Edition: **2023**

ISBN: 978-93-5465-751-1

Printed at: Sterling Graphics Pvt. Ltd. India.

PREFACE

The early clinical exposure (ECE) has been introduced in the 1st MBBS curriculum as a part of vertical integration between the first year and the final year subjects. According to Bloom's Taxonomy (cognitive domain, based on acquisition of knowledge) has been reclassified in 2001 as:

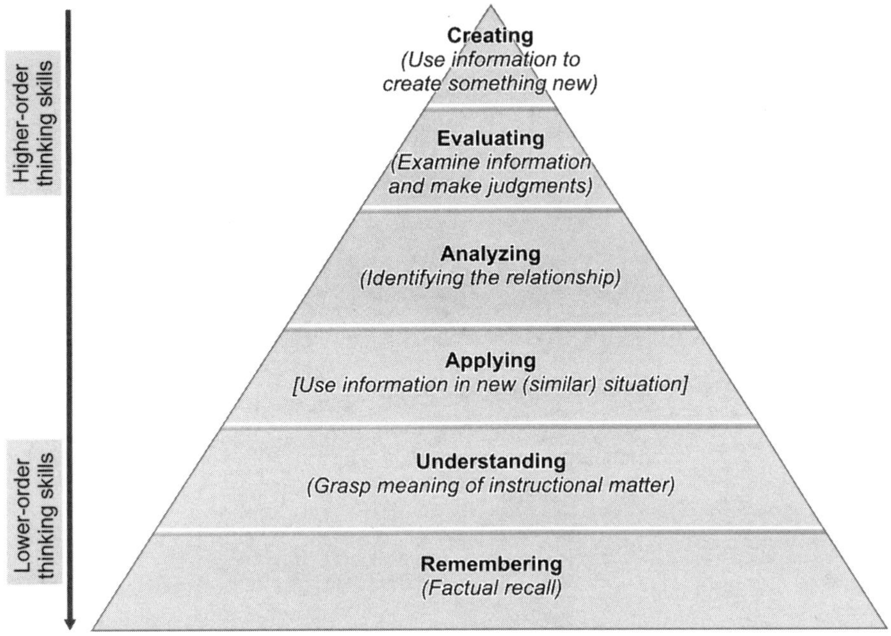

According to this, the learner has to atleast use the factual concepts in application of knowledge (level 3 of Bloom's taxonomy) during the First Professional MBBS. Hence, ECE provides a platform for easily attaining this level. Further, ECE gives a good exposure to the students, in gaining an insight into clinical and social aspects of patient care. In the second professional, the student gets to attend the clinics and starts applying the knowledge gained through the ECE chapters. Understanding the medicine through physiological basis of disease and its management will help the students to build a proper perspective that embraces the clinical content and helps them become a good medical professional and a competent Indian Medical Graduate.

Manjinder Kaur

ACKNOWLEDGMENTS

We acknowledge the inspiration and support of our students, colleagues and family in completion of this book.

We wish to thank Dr Rishi Sharma, Professor of Respiratory Medicine and Dr Pankaj Gupta, Consultant Gastroenterology for their help in constructing the clinical cases in Respiratory and Gastrointestinal Physiology respectively.

We also extend our gratitude towards whole team of M/s Jaypee Brothers Medical Publishers (P) Ltd, New Delhi, India, Shri Jitendar P Vij (Group Chairman), Mr Ankit Vij (Managing Director), Mr MS Mani (Group President), Dr Madhu Choudhary (Director–Educational Publishing), Ms Pooja Bhandari (Production Head), Ms Sunita Katla (Executive Assistant to Group Chairman and Publishing Manager), Ms Samina Khan (Executive Assistant to Director–Educational Publishing), Dr Aditya Tayal (Team Leader–UG Publishing), Mr Rajesh Sharma (Production Coordinator), Ms Seema Dogra (Cover Visualizer), Mr Narsingh Kumar (Proofreader), Mr Akshay Thakur (Typesetter), Mr Radhe Shyam Singh (Graphic Designer) for successful completion of this book.

CONTENTS

COMPETENCY TABLE

Number	COMPETENCY The student should be able to:	Core (Y/N)	Chapter number	Page number
PY2.5	Describe different types of anemias and jaundice.	Y	1	1–8
PY2.8	Describe the physiological basis of hemostasis and anticoagulants. Describe bleeding and clotting disorders (hemophilia, purpura).	Y	1	1–8
PY3.4	Describe the structure of neuromuscular junction and transmission of impulses.	Y	2	9–12
PY3.5	Discuss the action of neuromuscular blocking agents.	Y	2	9–12
PY3.6	Describe the pathophysiology of myasthenia gravis.	Y	2	9–12
PY3.13	Describe muscular dystrophy: Myopathies.	Y	2	9–12
PY4.9	Discuss the physiology aspects of: Peptic ulcer, gastroesophageal reflux disease, vomiting, diarrhea, constipation, adynamic ileus, Hirschsprung's disease.	Y	3	13–18
PY5.6	Describe abnormal ECG, arrhythmia, heart block and myocardial infarction.	Y	4	19–26
PY5.11	Describe the pathophysiology of shock, syncope and heart failure.	Y	4	19–26
PY6.5	Describe and discuss the principles of artificial respiration, oxygen therapy, acclimatization and decompression sickness.	Y	5	27–31
PY7.6	Describe the innervations of urinary bladder, physiology of micturition and its abnormalities.	Y	6	32–34
PY7.7	Describe artificial kidney, dialysis and renal transplantation.	Y	6	32–34
PY8.2	Describe the synthesis, secretion, transport, physiological actions, regulation and effect of altered (hypo and hyper) secretion of pituitary gland, thyroid gland, parathyroid gland, adrenal gland, pancreas and hypothalamus.	Y	7	35–48
PY8.4	Describe function tests: Thyroid gland, adrenal cortex, adrenal medulla and pancreas.	Y	7	35–48
PY9.1	Describe and discuss sex determination; sex differentiation and their abnormalities and outline psychiatry and practical implication of sex determination.	Y	11	66–68
PY9.8	Describe and discuss the physiology of pregnancy, parturition and lactation and outline the psychology and psychiatry-disorders associated with it.	Y	8	49–52
PY9.9	Interpret a normal semen analysis report including (a) sperm count, (b) sperm morphology and (c) sperm motility, as per WHO guidelines and discuss the results.	Y	8	49–52
PY9.10	Discuss the physiological basis of various pregnancy tests.	Y	8	49–52
PY9.12	Discuss the common causes of infertility in a couple and role of IVF in managing a case of infertility.	Y	8	49–52
PY10.6	Describe and discuss spinal cord, its functions, lesion and sensory disturbances.	Y	9	53–60
PY10.7	Describe and discuss functions of cerebral cortex, basal ganglia, thalamus, hypothalamus, cerebellum and limbic system and their abnormalities.	Y	9	53–60
PY10.9	Describe and discuss the physiological basis of memory, learning and speech.	Y	9	53–60

CHAPTER 1

Hematology

PY 2.5 Describe different types of anemia and jaundice.
PY 2.8 Describe the physiological basis of hemostasis and anticoagulants. Describe bleeding and clotting disorders (hemophilia, purpura).

LEARNING OBJECTIVES

After finishing this module, you should be able to:

- Analyze the clinical problem on the basis of its signs and symptoms, laboratory findings, to reach a differential diagnosis for that problem.
- Describe the pathophysiology of the given clinical condition based on the clinical and laboratory findings.
- Discuss the rationale of management, based on the derangement of physiological parameters in a case scenario.

CASE 1.1 IRON DEFICIENCY ANEMIA

A 35-year-old female complains of breathlessness, loss of appetite, apathy and easy fatiguability. Examination of the patient revealed pallor, koilonychia, increased heart rate and systolic murmur.

Laboratory investigations of this patient were obtained as under:

- **Hemoglobin:** 6.0 g% (Reference value: 12–14 g% in females; 14–16 g% in males)
- **Packed cell volume (PCV):** 30% (Reference value: 42–45%)
- **RBC count:** 3.0 million/cu.mm (Reference value: 4.5–5.5 million/cu.mm)
- **S. ferritin:** 9 nanogram/mL (Reference value: 12–300 ng/mL)
- **Mean corpuscular volume (MCV):** 70 fL (Reference value: 80–100 fL)
- **Total iron binding capacity (TIBC):** 500 microgram/dL (Reference value: 240–450 microgram/dL)
- **Mean corpuscular hemoglobin concentration (MCHC):** 28% (Reference value: 32–36%)
- **Peripheral blood film (PBF):** RBC are microcytic and hypochromic

Based on the above case, answer the following questions:

1. What do you think this patient is suffering from?
2. How would you grade the anemia of this patient based on clinical classification?
3. What do you understand about microcytic and hypochromic RBCs in this patient?
4. How is the deficient nutrient absorbed and utilized in our body?
5. Define anemia.
6. Classify anemia according to the etiology (cause).
7. Classify anemia according to the morphology of RBCs.
8. Describe the physiological basis of clinical features/symptoms of this disease.

Provisional diagnosis: Iron deficiency anemia (IDA).
Definition: Decreased oxygen carrying capacity of blood with or without decreased hemoglobin content or RBC count or both.

Classification of Anemia

Etiological Classification

Table 1.1: Etiological classification of anemia.

Main etiology	*Increased blood loss*		*Increased breakdown of RBC*				*Decreased production of RBC*	
Various causes	Acute blood loss	Chronic blood loss	Red cell membrane defects	Enzyme defects	Abnormal hemoglobin	Immune mediated hemolysis	Deficiency of nutrients	Bone marrow disorders
Examples	Acute hemorrhage due to road traffic accident, major surgeries, etc.	Hemorrhoids (piles), hookworm infestation, dysfunctional uterine bleeding in women, etc.	Hereditary spherocytosis, ovalocytosis	Glucose-6-phosphate dehydrogenase (G6PD) deficiency	Sickle cell anemia	Incompatible ABO blood transfusion	Iron deficiency, folic acid/vitamin B_{12} deficiency, protein deficiency	Aplastic anemia, etc.

Morphological Classification

Table 1.2: Morphological classification of anemia.

	Hypochromic (MCHC <31 g/dL)	*Normochromic (MCHC = 31–33 g/dL)*
Size of RBC <7 µm (microcytic; MCV <80 fL)	Iron deficiency anemia thalassemia lead poisoning	Chronic infection
Size of RBC = 7 µm (normocytic, MCV = 80–100 fL)	Chronic hemorrhage	• Acute blood loss hemolytic anemia • Aplastic anemia
Size of RBC >7 µm (macrocytic; MCV> 100 fL)	Liver disease	• Vitamin B_{12} deficiency • Folic acid deficiency

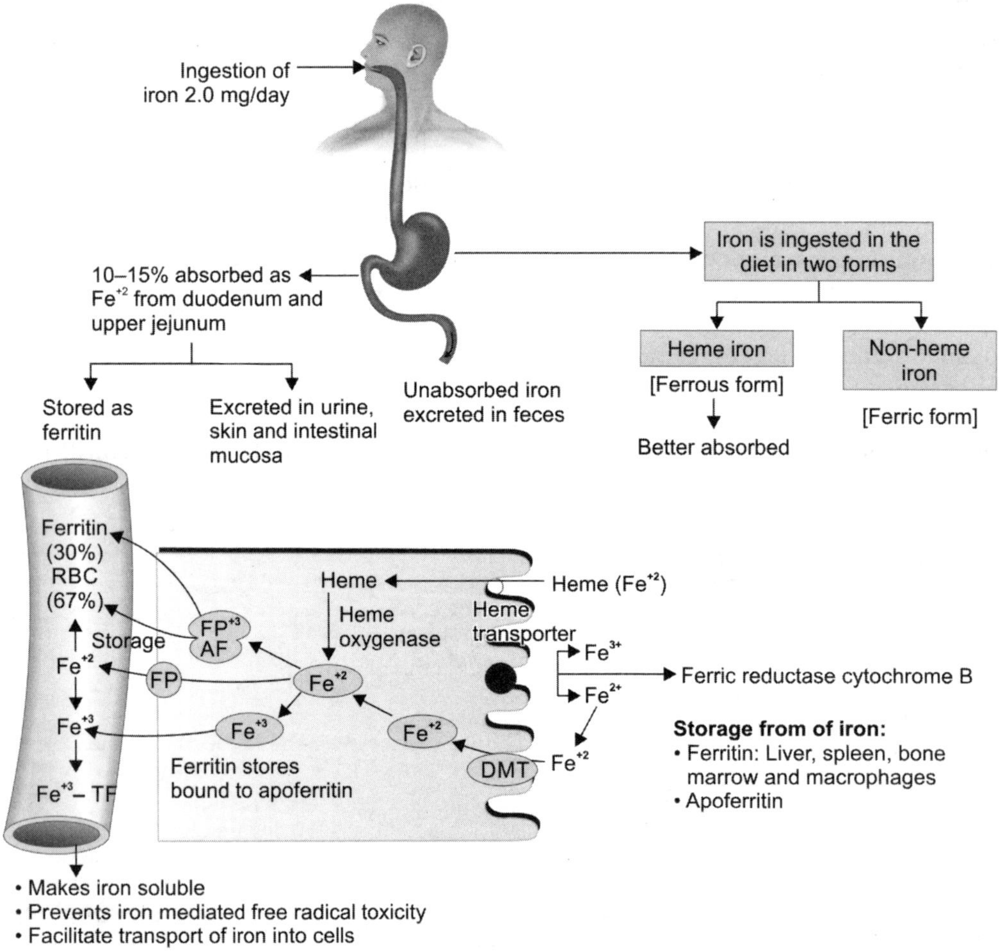

Fig. 1.1: Absorption of iron from GIT.

[DMT: divalent metal transporter; FP: ferro protein transporter; TF: trans ferritin (synthesized in the liver); AF: apoferritin]

Clinical Classification

Table 1.3: Clinical classification of anemia.

Concentration of Hb	*Grades of anemia*
>10 g/dL	No anemia
8–10 g/dL	Mild anemia
5–8 g/dL	Moderate anemia
<5 g/dL	Severe anemia

Absorption of Iron from GIT

Refer **Figure 1.1**.

Pathophysiology of IDA and Physiology of Clinical Symptoms (Fig. 1.2)

Lab Diagnosis

- Decreased RBC count (<4.5 million/cc in females and 5 million/cc in males) and hemoglobin content (<10 g/dL)
- Peripheral blood film shows microcytic hypochromic RBCs
- Red cell indices: MCV < 80fl, MCHC < 31g/dL
- Decreased S. ferritin levels (<10 ng/mL in adult females and <20 ng/mL in adult males)
- Increased total iron binding capacity (TIBC) (>450 mcg/mL)

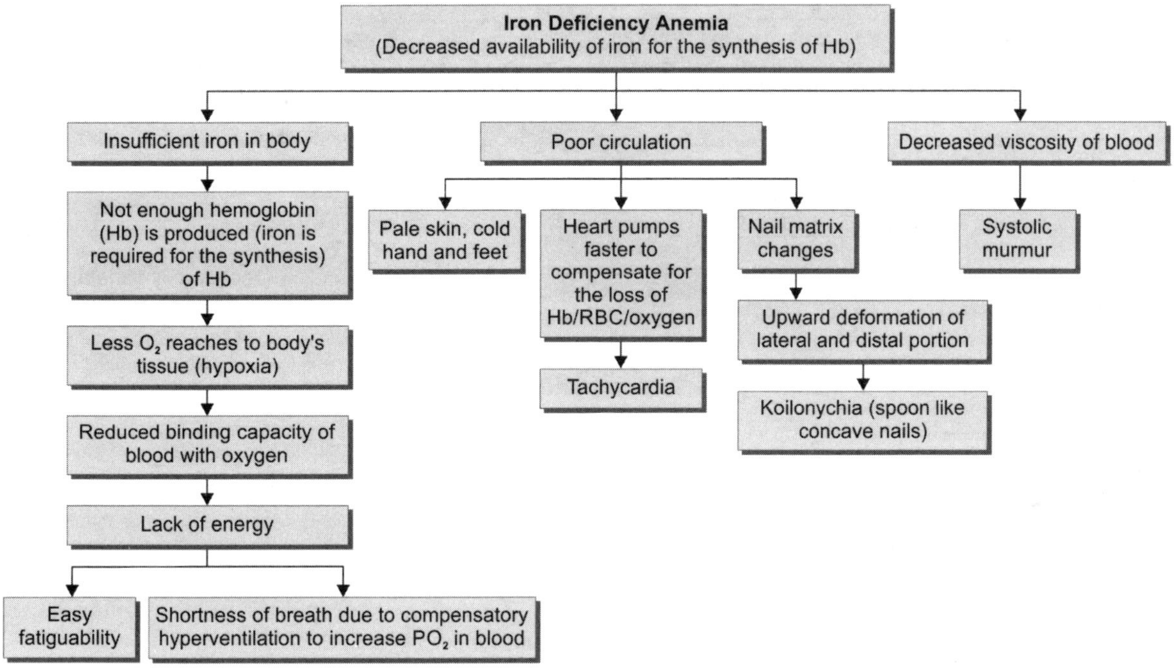

Fig. 1.2: Physiological basis of clinical features of iron deficiency anemia.

CASE 1.2 ANEMIA DUE TO VITAMIN B_{12} DEFICIENCY

A 45-year-old male complains of indigestion, diarrhea, soreness in angles of mouth, loss of appetite and tingling sensation in the hands and feet. Examination of the patient revealed angular stomatitis, red beefy tongue and peripheral neuropathy.

Lab investigations of these patients were obtained as under:

- **Hemoglobin:** 9.0 g%
- **RBC count:** 1 million/cu.mm.
- **S. Iron:** 170 microgram/dL (Reference value: 60–170 mg/dL)
- **MCV:** 100 fL
- **MCH:** 50 pg
- **Reticulocyte count:** 6% (Reference value: 1–2%)

Based on the above case, answer the following questions:

1. What do you think this patient is suffering from?
2. What is the cause of peripheral neuropathy in this type of anemia?
3. Why do you see large nucleated RBC (megaloblasts) in PBF, in this condition?
4. How is the deficient nutrient absorbed and utilized in our body?
5. Why is this type of anemia seen in patients with gastric atrophy?
6. What are the other conditions with a similar blood picture? What are the causes for the same?
7. What will happen if you give only folic acid supplementation in pernicious anemia?

PBF: RBC are macrocytic and normochromic with some large nucleated RBC, neutropenia with hypersegmented neutrophils and decreased platelets per high power field.

Provisional diagnosis: Megaloblastic anemia (vitamin B_{12} deficiency).

> **Note:** Deficiency of intrinsic factor due to autoimmune causes is termed as pernicious anemia

Absorption of Vitamin B_{12} from GIT (*Refer* Figure 1.3)

Both Vitamin B_{12} and folic acid, act as methyl carriers and are responsible for the nuclear maturation of the cells, hence present with macrocytic, normochromic and megaloblastic anemia. The cytoplasmic maturation of the cells is normal.

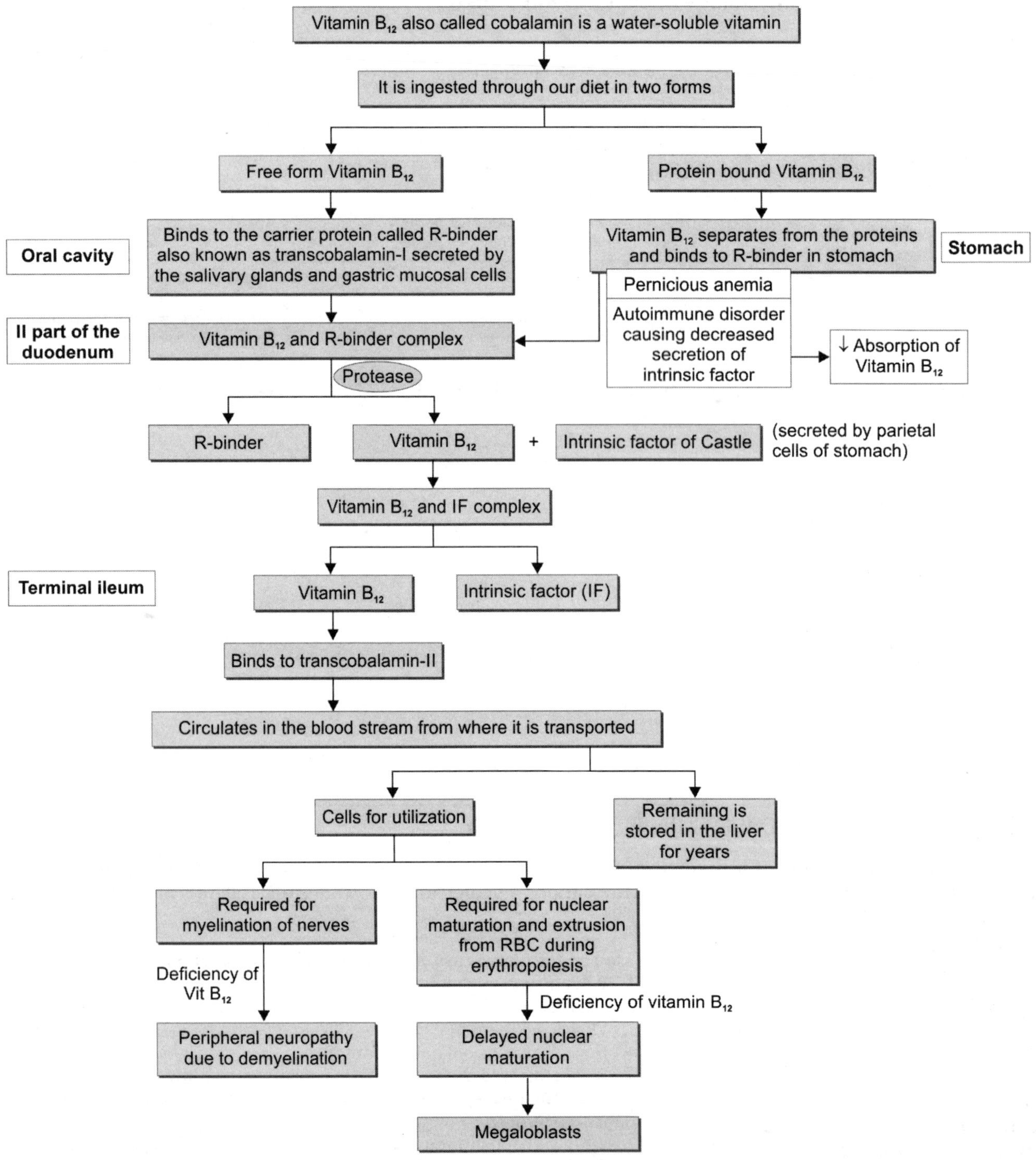

Fig. 1.3: Absorption of vitamin B_{12} from GIT.

Table 1.4: Various causes of vitamin B_{12} deficiency.		
	Gastric	*Intestinal*
Cause	Deficiency of intrinsic factor (IF)	Decrease absorption of vitamin B_{12}
Examples	• Autoimmune causes of failure of secretion of IF (pernicious anemia) • Gastrectomy • Congenital lack of IF	• Tropical sprue • Crohn's disease • Fish tapeworm infestation • Intestinal blind loop syndrome

Supplementation of only folic acid, in a patient with vitamin B_{12} deficiency, may result in improvement of blood picture but worsening of peripheral neuropathy. Hence, the patient should be properly evaluated before starting the supplementation.

PBF: The RBCs in peripheral blood film of megaloblastic anemia (both in vitamin B_{12} and folic acid deficiency) are macrocytic and normochromic. The red cells are larger in size but the hemoglobin concentration is normal (increased MCV, normal MCHC). Some of the RBCs are nucleated (seive like nucleus) ; called as megaloblasts, hence the name ***'megaloblastic anemia'***. The other cells (WBCs and platelets) are also affected showing neutropenia and shift to right on Cooke-Arneth along with thrombocytopenia.

Various causes of vitamin B_{12} deficiency are given in **Table 1.4**.

CASE 1.3 G-6-PD DEFICIENCY: HEMOLYTIC ANEMIA

A 20-year-old male complains of pain in loin and passage of dark urine after eating fava beans. Examination of the patient revealed nothing significant.

Lab investigations of this patient were obtained as under:

- **Hemoglobin:** 10 g%
- **RBC count:** 3 million/cu.mm.

(***Note:*** Plasma hemoglobin and methemoglobin levels are raised)

PBF: RBC are normocytic and normochromic with polychromasia, basophilic stipplings and marked poikilocytosis.

Based on the above case, answer the following questions:

1. What do you think this patient is suffering from?
2. What are the causes of this type of anemia?
3. What is the mechanism of action of the deficient enzyme in this condition?
4. How can you prevent this condition?
5. What are the other types of hemolytic anemia and what is the cause in each one of them?
6. What are target cells? In which condition, they are seen?

Provisional diagnosis: Hemolytic anemia (G-6-PD deficiency).
Hemolytic anemia could occur due to many causes, as given in **Table 1.5**.

Table 1.5: Causes of hemolytic anemia.	
Due to defects within the RBCs (intracorpuscular defects)	*Due to various pathologies outside the RBCs (extracorpuscular defects)*
Defects in red cell membrane: • Hereditary spherocytosis • Hereditary ovalocytosis	Mechanical trauma to RBCs: • Thrombi within circulation • Exotoxins
Defective hemoglobin chains (hemoglobinopathies): • Thalassemia • Sickle cell anemia	Antigen antibody mediated hemolysis: • ABO incompatibility • Rh incompatibility • Drug induced
Enzyme defects: • G-6 PD deficiency • Pyruvate kinase and hexokinase deficiency	

Pathophysiology of G-6-PD Deficiency and Physiology of Clinical Symptoms

See **Figure 1.4**.

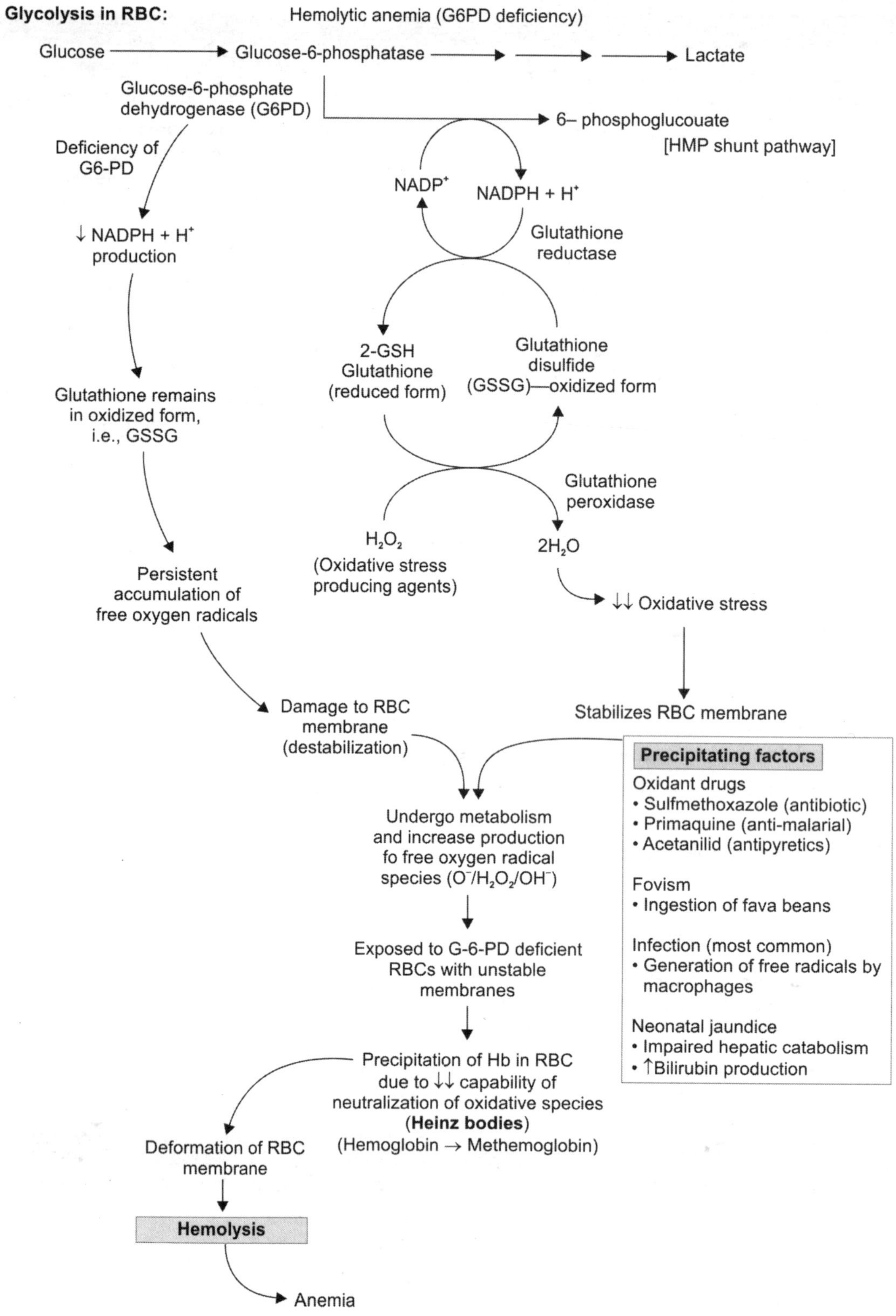

Fig. 1.4: Pathophysiology of G-6-PD deficiency anemia.

CASE 1.4 ERYTHROBLASTOSIS FETALIS

A 4-day-old home delivered male baby was brought to the pediatrician with complaints of excessive cry and jaundice. The mother of the baby is from a village and did not avail any ante-natal check-up during the pregnancy. She has a 2-year-old male child who was a full term normal home delivered baby.

Mother has no H/o abortion and no H/o jaundice in the first baby after birth. Details of the blood group of the family are not available.

On examination: Baby is lethargic with poor muscle tone, poor feeding and jaundice.

Investigations:

- **Mother:** Blood group is B negative.
- **Baby:**
  - *Blood group:* AB positive
  - *Hb:* 10 g%
  - Erythroblasts: Abundant (erythroblastemia)
  - *S. bilirubin:* 18 mg/dL (Reference value: 0.2-0.8 mg/dL)

Based on the above clinical scenario answer the following questions:

1. What is the probable diagnosis?
2. What is the pathophysiology behind the clinical condition presented?
3. How can this condition be prevented in subsequent pregnancies?
4. What is the physiological basis of prophylaxis given?

Provisional diagnosis: Hemolytic disease of newborn due to Rh incompatibility (erythroblastosis fetalis).

Pathophysiology of hemolytic disease of newborn (HDN) (Fig. 1.5)

The first pregnancy can also be affected by Rh incompatibility, in case of previous exposure to D-antigen (as in case of transfusion of Rh positive blood to Rh negative lady).

The concentration of anti-D antibodies formed in the mother will depend upon the antigen load entering the maternal circulation.

Based on the severity of HDN, it is classified as:

1. **Hydrops fetalis:** Most severe. Baby is swollen and baby dies in utero or few hours after birth.
2. **Icterus gravis neonatorum:** Characterized by hemolytic jaundice, anemia, erythroblastemia, kernicterus (deposition of bilirubin in basal ganglia, if more than 18 g%) and liver damage.

Prophylaxis: Inj. Anti-D (RhoGam) within 72 hours of delivery. It is a type of passive immunity.

Treatment:

1. Intrauterine fetal blood transfusion
2. Exchange transfusion: Transfusing Rh negative blood of same ABO type to stop hemolysis, till the antibodies persist in neonatal blood.
3. Phototherapy
4. Immunoglobulin therapy

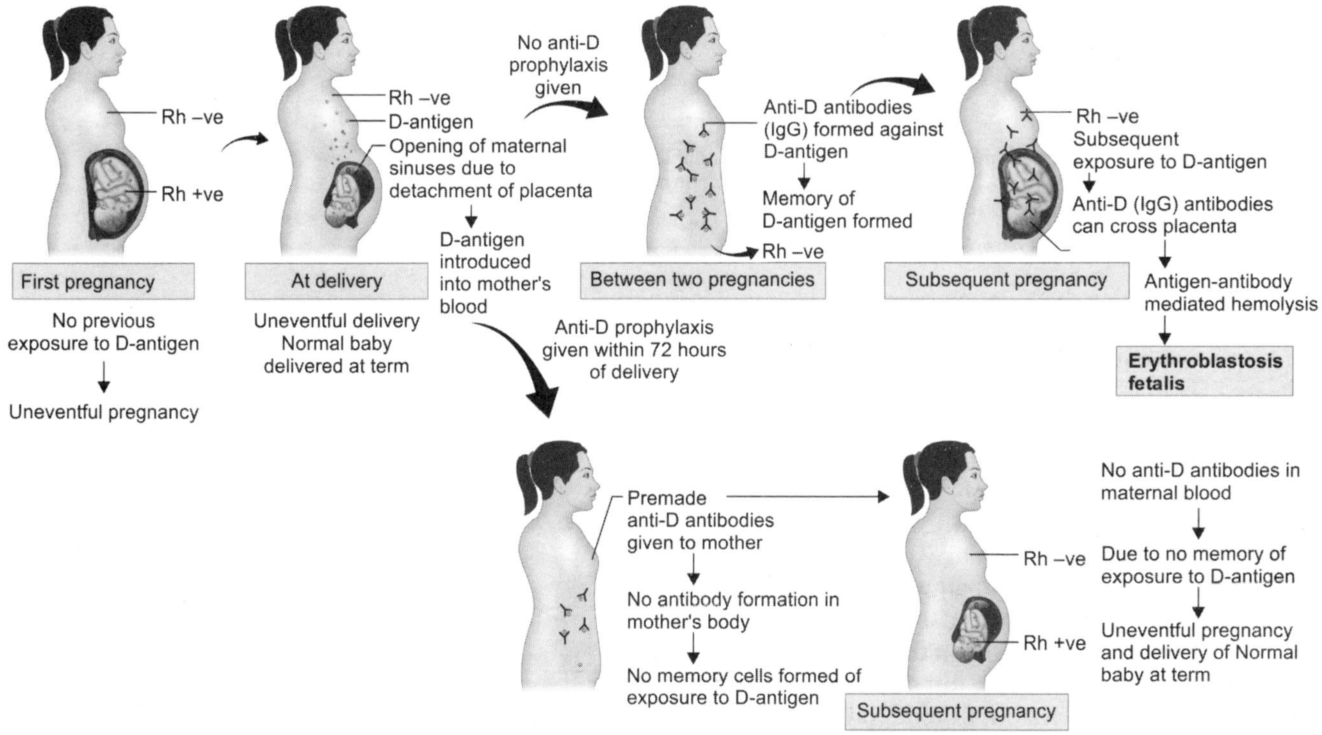

Fig. 1.5: Pathophysiology of hemolytic disease of newborn.

CASE 1.5 HEMOPHILIA

A young boy of 8-year-old complained of a swollen knee after he fell from the bicycle. He also complained of some bluish discoloration of the skin of right arm. His past history is suggestive of prolonged bleeding even after minor injury. On examination he was found to have a hematoma of the knee. His lab investigations show prolonged CT, APTT with normal BT and PT. His hemoglobin is 9.0 g%.

Based on the above clinical scenario answer the following questions:
1. What is the probable diagnosis?
2. Why is the bleeding time normal in this patient despite a prolonged CT and APTT?
3. What is the physiological basis of the clinical symptoms?

Provisional diagnosis: Hemophilia A
Hemophilia is a bleeding disorder and is of two types:
1. **Hemophilia A:** Due to deficiency of factor VIII (more common)
2. **Hemophilia B:** Due to deficiency of factor IX

Hemophilia A is a clinical condition that arises due to deficiency of factor VIII resulting in bleeding tendencies.

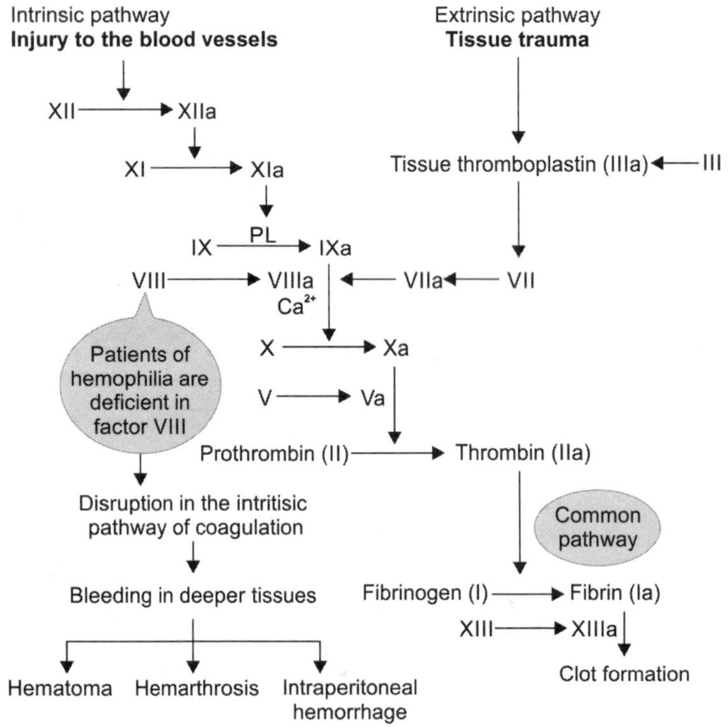

Fig. 1.6: Pathophysiology of hemophilia A.
(PL: phospholipid)

Factor VIII is present on the X- chromosome and hence it is inherited as a X-linked recessive genetic disorder.

Diagnosis of hemophilia begins with a good clinical history and physical examination supported by the following laboratory investigations:
1. **Bleeding time (BT):** Normal (as platelet count is normal, temporary hemostasis is not affected).
2. **Clotting time (CT):** Prolonged (due to derangement in the intrinsic pathway of coagulation).
3. **Prothrombin time (PT):** Normal X
   - PT is a test used for extrinsic pathway and common pathway of coagulation (factors involved are VII, X, V, II, I)
4. **Activated partial thromboplastin time (APTT):** Prolonged.
   - Test is used for intrinsic and common pathway of coagulation (factors involved are XII, XI, IX, VIII, X, V, II, I)
   - Factor VIII and IX are a part of intrinsic pathway, so APTT is increased in hemophilia A and hemophilia B).

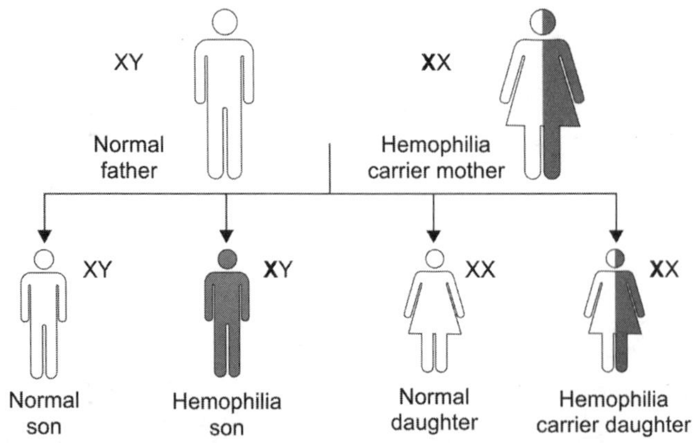

Fig. 1.7: Inheritance in hemophilia A patients.

2 CHAPTER Musculoskeletal Physiology

PY 3.4 Describe the structure of neuromuscular junction and transmission of impulses.
PY 3.5 Discuss the action of neuromuscular blocking agents.
PY 3.6 Describe the pathophysiology of myasthenia gravis.
PY 3.13 Describe muscular dystrophy: Myopathies.

LEARNING OBJECTIVES

After finishing this module, you should be able to:
- Analyze the clinical problem on the basis of its signs and symptoms, laboratory findings, to reach a differential diagnosis for that problem.
- Describe the pathophysiology of the given clinical condition based on the clinical and laboratory findings.
- Discuss the rationale of management, based on the derangement of physiological parameters in a case scenario.

CASE 2.1 MYASTHENIA GRAVIS

History: A 25-year-old lady comes to OPD with chief complaints of weakness and fatigability. Generally, during morning she does not feel any significant weakness but, as day passes and she gets involved in routine household works, weakness gradually starts to increase. The condition improves by some rest or sleep. She also reports double vision and difficulty in swallowing.

Physical examination: Ptosis, diplopia, proximal muscle weakness, normal deep tendon reflex, no sensory impairment.

Lab Investigations

- Positive anticholinesterase test
- Electrodiagnostic testing shows rapid reduction in amplitude of the repetitive nerve stimulation (decremental response).

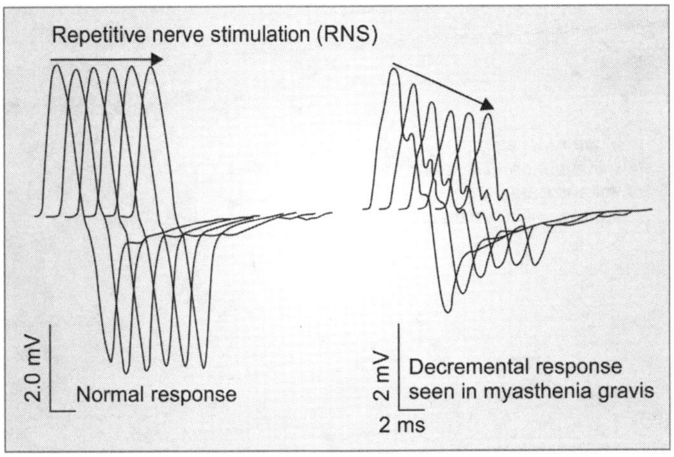

Fig. 2.1: Electrodiagnostic repetitive nerve stimulation.

Based on above clinical condition, answer the following questions:
1. What do you think this patient is suffering from?
2. As the day passes, why does the patient gradually start to get more and more fatigue?
3. Why does rest improve the symptoms?
4. Why does the subject have diplopia and ptosis?
5. How do you interpret the electrodiagnostic finding?
6. What could be the physiological basis of management?
7. What is the pathology in Lambert-Eaton syndrome? How is it different from myasthenia gravis?

Provisional Diagnosis

Myasthenia gravis.

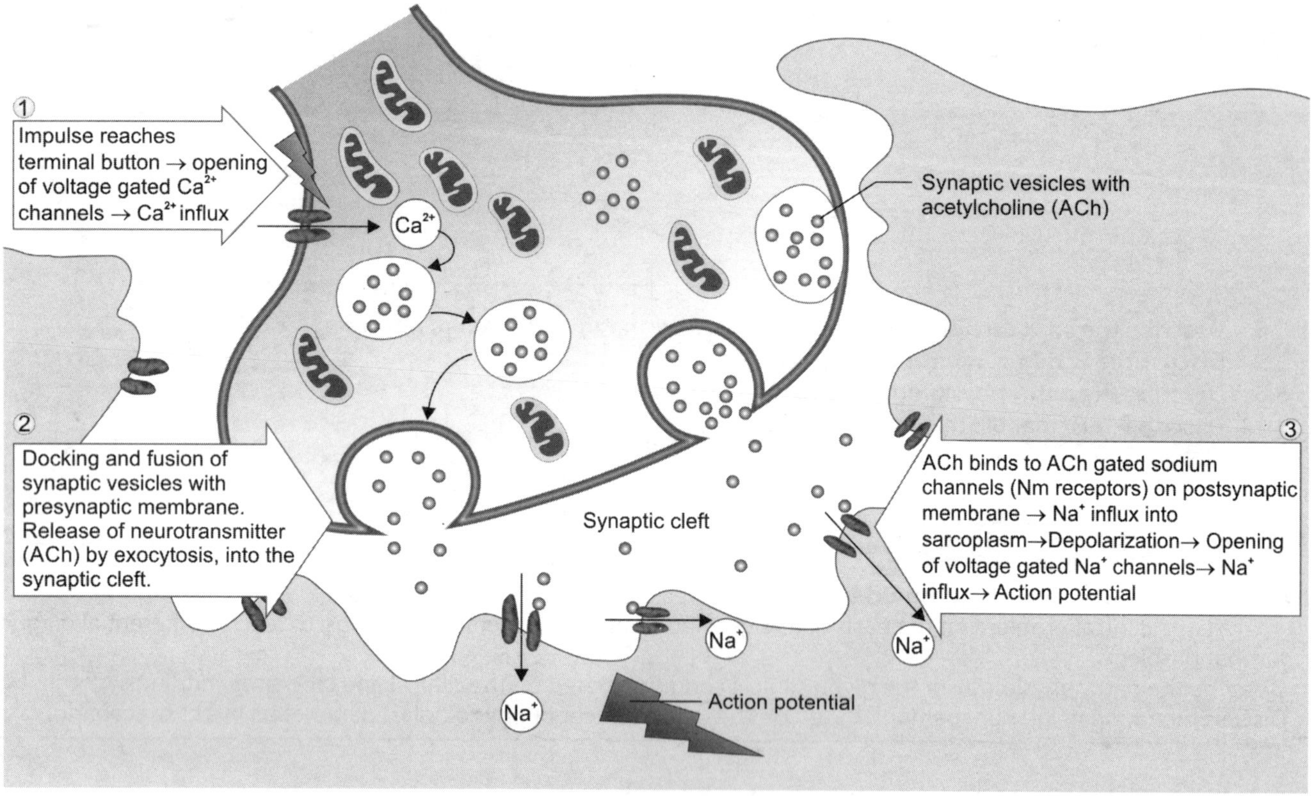

Fig. 2.2: Healthy neuromuscular junction showing transmission of impulse.

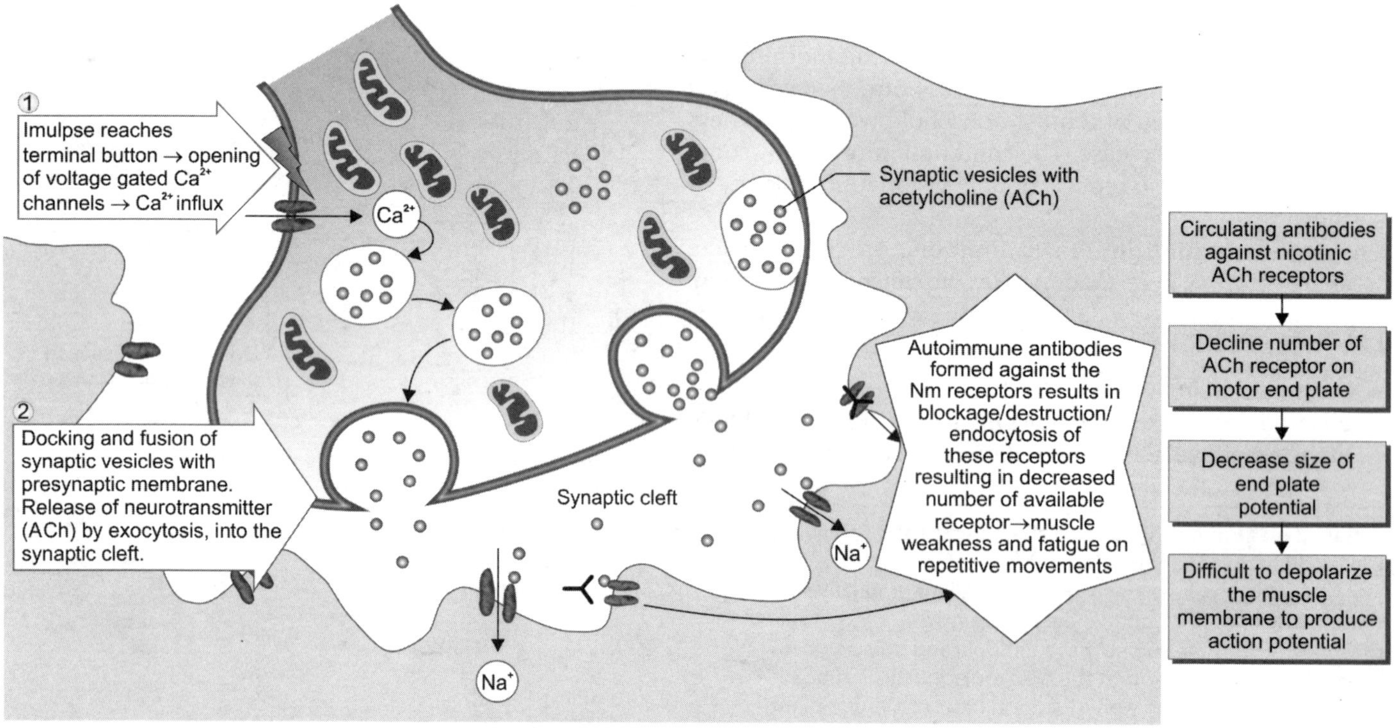

Fig. 2.3: Pathophysiology of myasthenia gravis.

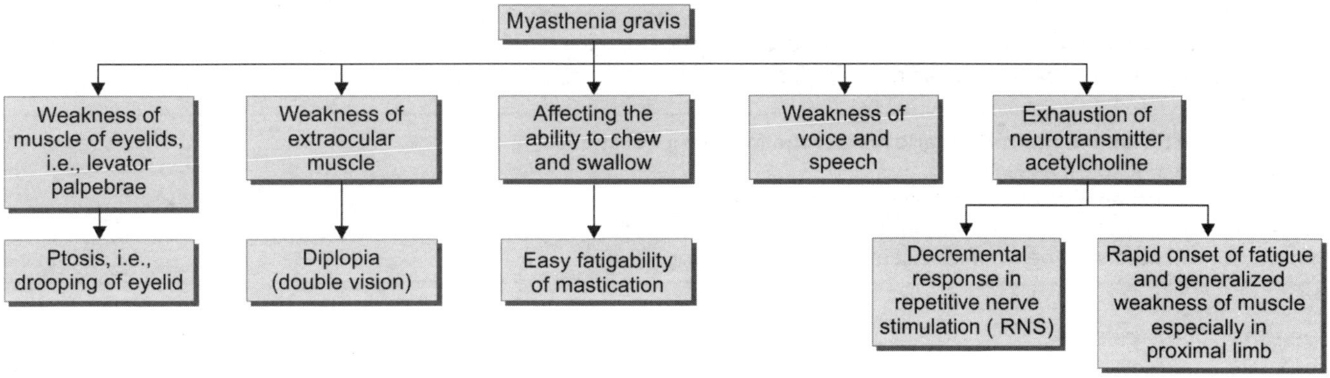

Fig. 2.4: Clinical features in myasthenia gravis patients.

Hence, the patient of MG, feels weakness on repetitive movements due to exhaustion of neurotransmitter but his symptoms improve on rest (due to resynthesis of ACh).

Physiology of Management

Anticholinesterase Drugs (Neostigmine)

The ACh, released into the synaptic cleft has a very short half life. The acetylcholine is broken down by the enzyme acetylcholinesterase into acetyl-CoA and choline. Hence, if this enzyme is blocked the half life of acetylcholine increases in the synaptic cleft which increases its availability for the transmission of impulse across the neuromuscular junction improving the clinical symptoms of myasthenia gravis.

Lambert-Eaton Syndrome

The repetitive movements/stimuli result in improvement of muscle weakness due to accumulation of neurotransmitter. Hence, the repetitive nerve stimulation test shows an '***incremental response***'.

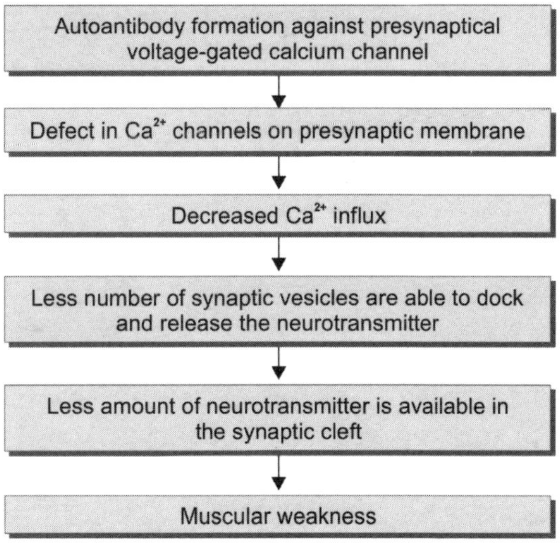

Fig. 2.5: Pathophysiology of Lambert-Eaton syndrome.

CASE 2.2 DUCHENNE MUSCULAR DYSTROPHY

An 8-year-old boy was brought to the pediatrician by the mother who complained that the child has frequent falls and has trouble running and climbing stairs for 2 years. The child finds difficulty in standing up from sitting posture now. The weakness is progressing gradually, since first noticed.

No history suggestive of any other significant medical or surgical illness in the past.

On Examination

- Child has a waddling gait
- Difficulty in jumping on the examination table

- Hypertrophied calf muscles
- Proximal muscle weakness of the pectoral and pelvic girdle muscles
- **Lab findings:** High S. creatine kinase and aldolase levels.

On the basis of the above clinical scenario answer the following questions:

1. What is the probable diagnosis?
2. What is the pathophysiology of the given condition?
3. What is the cause of high S.creatine kinase in this patient?
4. Why do you observe hypertrophied calf muscles in the patient?

Provisional Diagnosis

Duchenne muscular dystrophy.

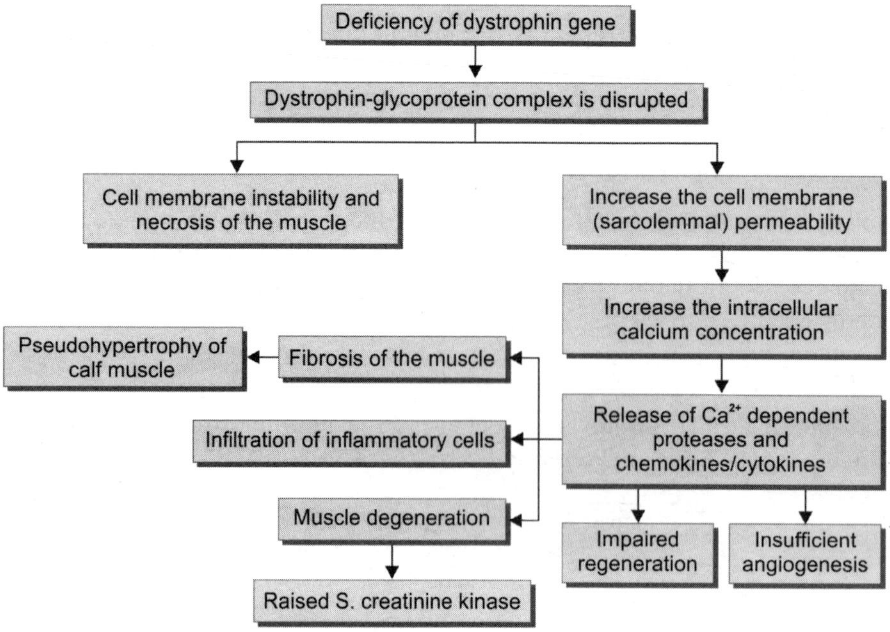

Fig. 2.6: Pathophysiology and clinical features of Duchenne muscular dystrophy.

3 CHAPTER Gastrointestinal System

PY 4.9 **Discuss the physiological aspects of peptic ulcer, gastroesophageal reflux disease (GERD), vomiting, diarrhea, constipation, adynamic ileus, Hirschsprung's disease.**

LEARNING OBJECTIVES

After finishing this module, you should be able to:

- Analyze the clinical problem on the basis of its signs and symptoms, laboratory findings, to reach a differential diagnosis for that problem.
- Describe the pathophysiology of the given clinical condition based on the clinical and laboratory findings.
- Discuss the rationale of management, based on the derangement of physiological parameters in a case scenario.

CASE 3.1 ACID PEPTIC DISEASE

A 35-year-old woman visits your OPD with chief complaints of pain in epigastrium which increase after taking food.

- **Past history:** Frequent intake of painkillers for her headache.
- Examination reveals no other significant finding

Based on the above case, answer the following questions:

1. What is your provisional diagnosis?
2. What are the probable causes for her problem?
3. How is this problem prevented in healthy individuals
4. What is post prandial alkaline tide?
5. What is the rationale for managing this case?

- **Provisional diagnosis:** Acid peptic disease.
- **Definition:** Peptic ulcer is a lesion in the mucosa of the digestive tract caused by the disruption of the mucosal integrity of the stomach and/or the duodenum.

Pathophysiology

- Under physiological limits there is a balance between the gastric acid secretion and gastroduodenal mucosal defense mechanism.
- Mucosal injury results when there is a disruption between the normal protective and precipitating mechanisms listed above.

Causes: Excessive use of ***non-steroidal anti-inflammatory drugs*** **(NSAIDs)** and ***Helicobacter pylori*** **infection** are the two major causes of peptic ulcer disease.

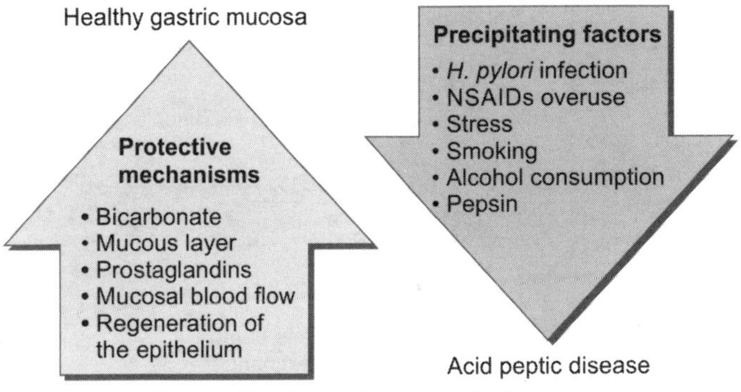

Fig. 3.1: Etiology of acid peptic disease.

Table 3.1: Difference between gastric ulcer and duodenal ulcer.

Gastric ulcer	*Duodenal ulcer*
Age: 50-60 years	30-40 years
Sex: More common in males	Sex: More common in the males
Pain: Epigastrium radiating to the back	Epigastrium
Onset: Immediately after meals	3–4 hours after meals or midnight
Aggravated: Food	Fasting
Relieved: Fasting or vomiting or lying down	By taking food
Appetite: Bad	Good
Weight loss: Present	Absent
Complications: • Hemorrhage presenting as hematemesis and melena • Perforation • Strictures	• **Complications:** • Hemorrhage presenting as hematemesis, melena • Perforation • Strictures

Investigations

- **Complete blood count:** To look for blood loss anemia.
- **Stool examination:** Evidence of melena (bleeding in the stools resulting in black and tarry stool).
- Upper gastrointestinal/esophagogastroduodenoscopy or endoscopy is diagnostic.

Physiology of Management

- **Lifestyle modification:**
  - Physical activity
  - Less consumption of oily, spicy, fried foods, tea and coffee
  - Stress management
- **Antisecretory drugs:** *Refer* **Fig 3.2A and B**.
  - *Antacids:* Acid neutralizing drugs containing magnesium or aluminium salts.
  - H_2 receptor antagonist (histamine receptor blockers: Ranitidine family).
  - Proton pump inhibitors (blocks H^+- K^+ ATPase pump in the parietal cells of gastric glands: Omeprazole).
  - *Ulcer-protective agents:* They coat the ulcer crater and prevent it from further damage and helps in healing: Surface coating drugs (mechanical barrier: Sucralfate).
  - Prostaglandin analogues.

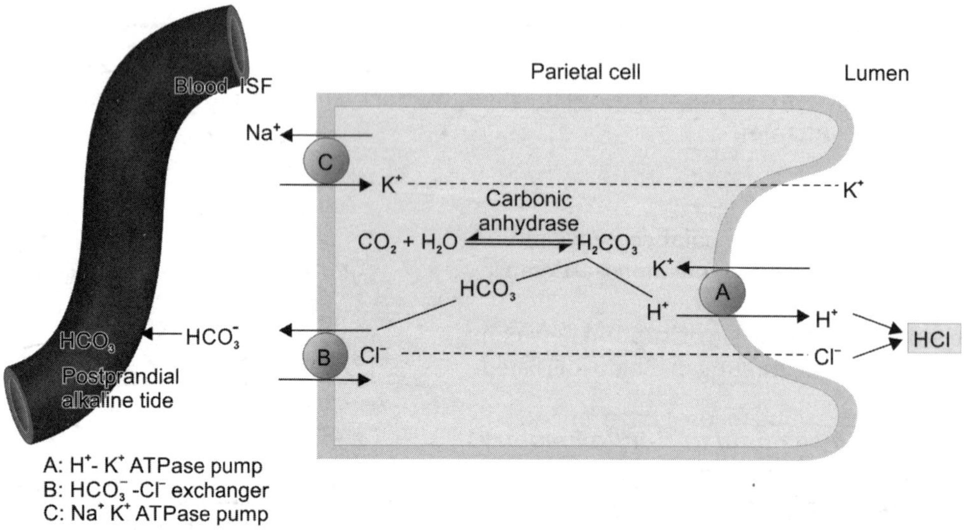

Fig. 3.2A: Mechanism of secretion of HCl.

(ISF: interstitial fluid)

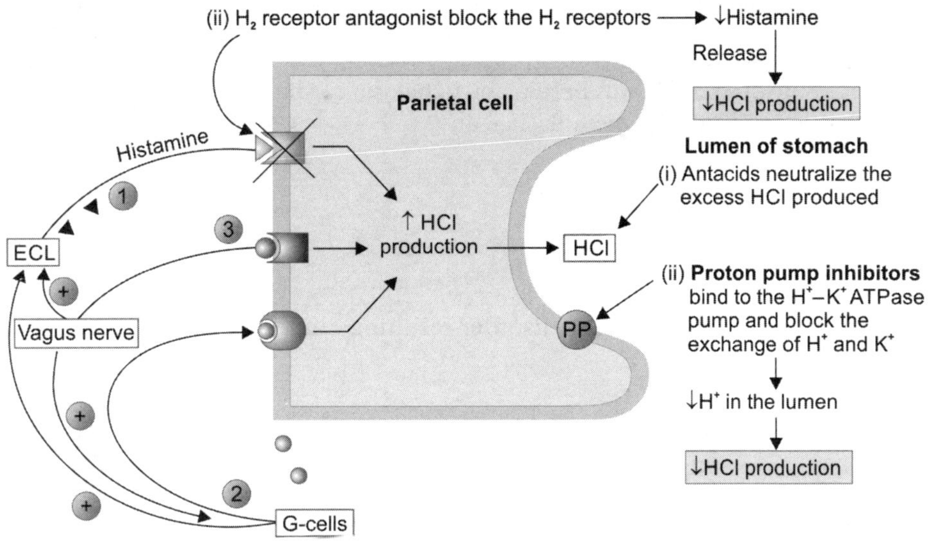

Fig. 3.2B: Mechanism of action of antisecretory agents.
(ECL: enterochromaffin-like cell)

CASE 3.2 GASTROESOPHAGEAL REFLUX DISEASE (GERD)

A 52-year-old man presents with complaints of retrosternal burning, regurgitation of food and retrosternal pain for the past 4 months. The symptoms have worsened now specially after a heavy meal and on lying down. He has no complaints of difficulty in swallowing or weight loss.

The patient has been taking a proton pump inhibitor (PPI) regularly over the past 12 weeks with partial resolution of his symptoms. No significant medical or surgical history in the past. He is a non-smoker with occasional alcohol intake.

On Examination

Patient is Obese

- **Vitals:** Normal
- **GPE:** Normal
- **CVS and abdominal system examination:** Normal.

> **Based on the above clinical scenario answer the following questions:**
> 1. What is the most likely diagnosis?
> 2. What is the physiological basis of symptoms of this disease?

Provisional diagnosis: Gastroesophageal reflux disease (GERD).

Definition: It is defined as a clinical condition that arises due to the backflow or regurgitation of the gastric contents into the esophagus which is anatomically not designed to withstand the acidic contents leading to local inflammation of the esophagus, i.e., esophagitis due to loss of tone of the lower esophageal sphincter (LES).

Pathophysiology

See **Figure 3.3**.

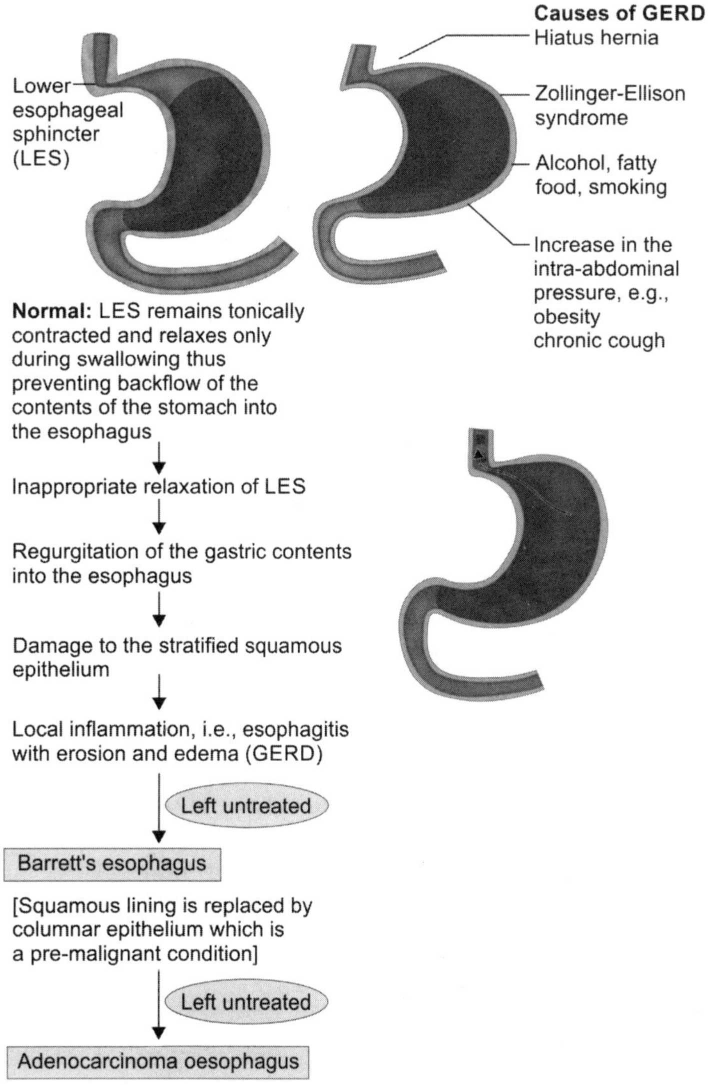

Fig. 3.3: Pathophysiology of GERD.

Investigations

- 24-hour pH monitoring in the lower esophagus
- Barium swallow to differentiate between hiatus hernia and achalasia cardia.
- Endoscopy and biopsy to rule out epithelial metaplasia if any.

Management

- Lifestyle modification
- Antacids and proton-pump inhibitors (temporary relief)
- Anti-reflux surgeries, e.g., fundoplication.

Achalasia cardia: Is a primary esophageal motility disorder resulting due to an increased tone of the lower esophageal sphincter (LES).

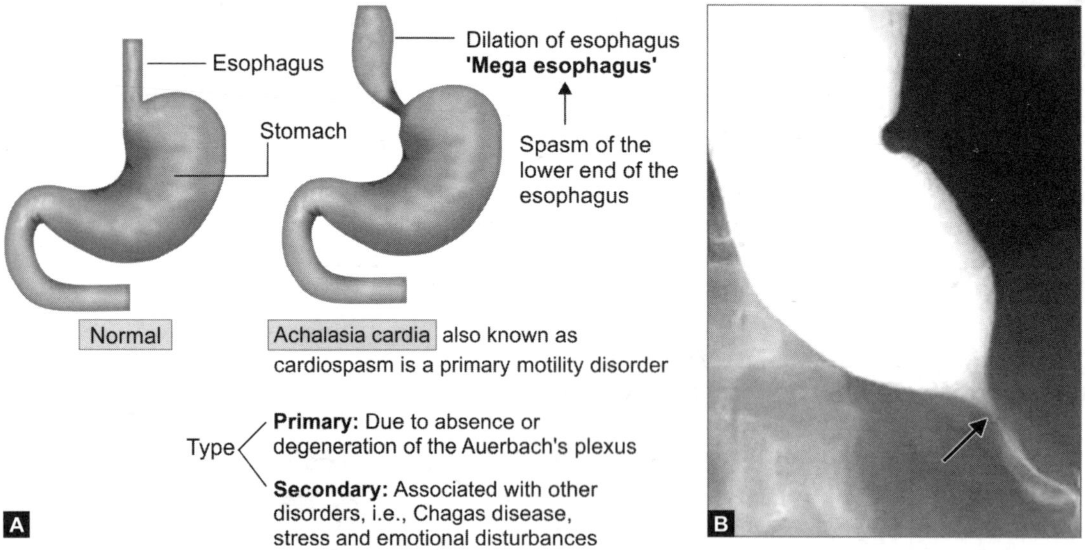

Figs. 3.4A and B: (A) Pathophysiology of achalasia cardia; (B) Barium swallow shows bird beak appearance.

CASE 3.3 OBSTRUCTIVE JAUNDICE

A 43-year-old female complains of:

a. Yellowish discoloration of eyes since 7 days

b. Pain in right hypochondrium which is radiating to right shoulder since 7 days

c. Fever since 2 days

On Examination

- Yellowish discoloration of sclera and mucous membrane
- Radiating pain to the right shoulder on palpating the right hypochondrium (Murphy's sign)

Laboratory Investigations

- Serum bilirubin—6 mg/dL (Reference value: <1.2 mg/dL)
- S. conjugated bilirubin—5 mg/dL (Reference value: <0.3 mg/dL)
- S. unconjugated bilirubin—1 mg/dL (Reference value: 0.2–0.8 mg/dL)
- SGOT—113 IU (3–4 times the upper normal limit)
- SGPT—110 IU (3–4 time the upper normal limit)
- Serum alkaline phosphatase—300 IU (3 times upper normal limit)

USG: Gallbladder is distended with distal acoustic shadowing and sludge. Common bile duct appears to be dilated.

Provisional diagnosis: Post-hepatic/obstructive/cholestatic jaundice.

Based on the above clinical scenario, answer the following questions:

1. What is your provisional diagnosis?
2. a. What is the role of liver function tests in differentiating the different type of jaundice?
   b. What is the importance of measuring conjugated and unconjugated bilirubin?
   c. What is the importance of measuring SGOT, SGPT and serum alkaline phosphatase?
3. What are the causes of different types of jaundice?
4. Describe the pathophysiology of jaundice.

Jaundice is defined as a clinical condition characterized by yellowish discoloration of the sclera, skin and mucous membrane known as icterus resulting from an increased bilirubin concentration (hyperbilirubinemia) in the body fluids. Clinically jaundice is detectable when the S. bilirubin exceeds 2–3 mg/100 mL. Obstruction to the bile flow due to any cause from hepatocytes to duodenum, i.e., (stone or tumor) causes cholestatic or obstructive or post hepatic jaundice.

Pathophysiology of Obstructive Jaundice

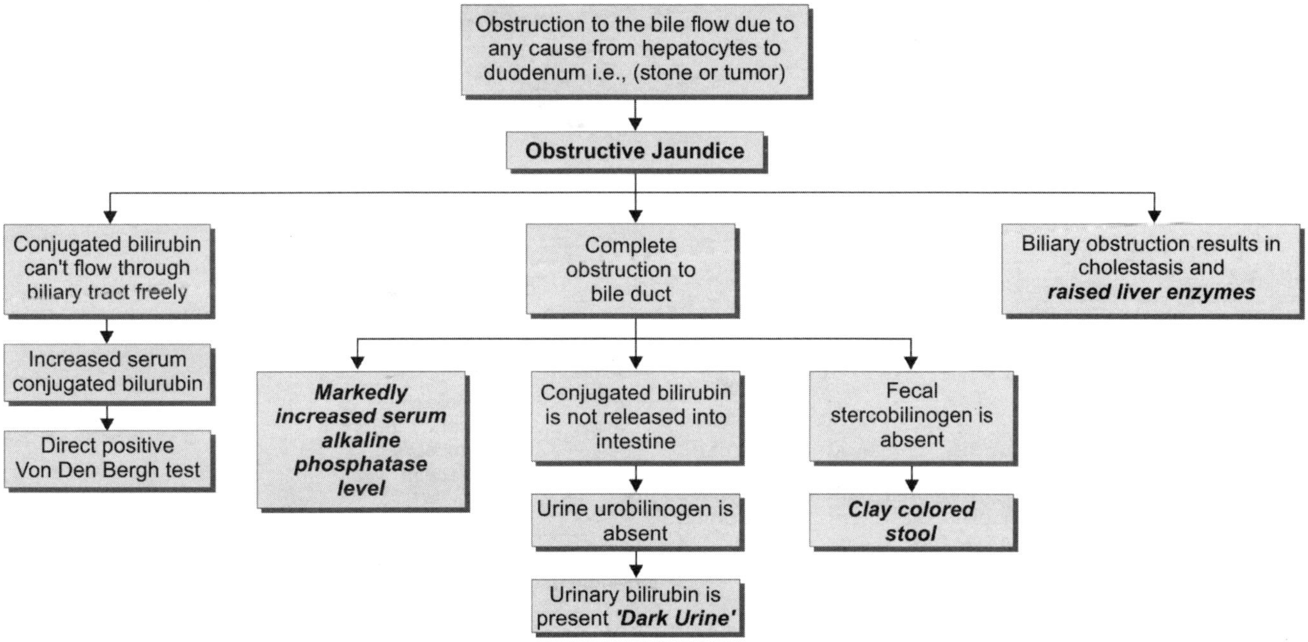

Fig. 3.5: Features of obstructive jaundice.

CASE 3.4 HIRSCHSPRUNG'S DISEASE

A 2-month-old male child was brought to the pediatrician with complaints of abdominal distension, constipation and excessive crying since 2 days.

On Examination

Distended abdomen with hard masses palpable.

- **Per Rectal Examination:**
    - Empty rectum
    - Hard fecal mass palpable

Investigation

- **Barium meal:** Small recutm with dilatation of the colon above the narrowed segment
- **Full thickness biopsy:** To demonstrate nerve plexus and confirm the absence of ganglionic cells.

Based on the above clinical scenario, answer the following questions:

1. What is the probable diagnosis?
2. What is the physiological basis of the symptoms of the disease?
3. What is the role of enteric nervous system in maintaining GI motility?

Provisional diagnosis: Hirschsprung disease/aganglionic megacolon.

Pathophysiology

Management: Resection of the affected segment.

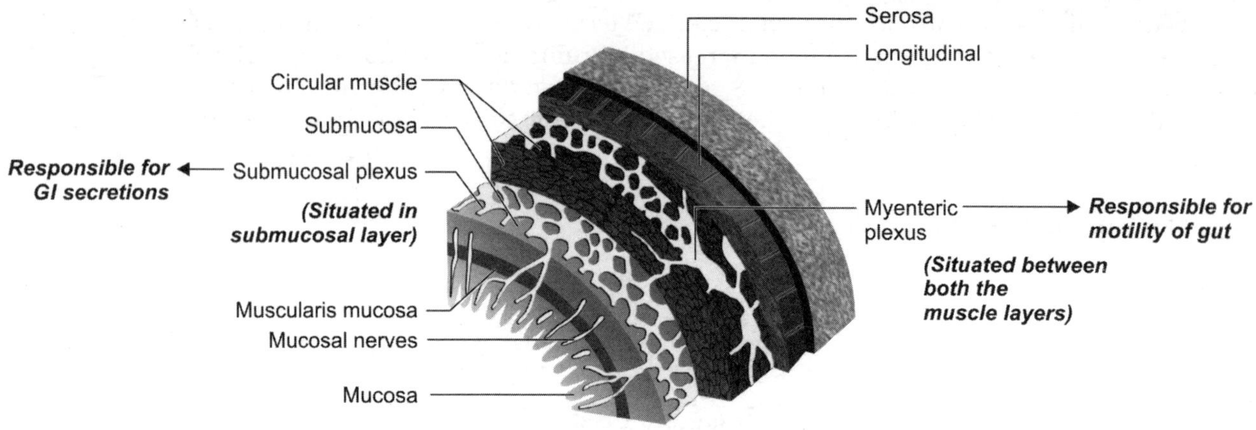

Fig. 3.6: Organization of GIT showing enteric nervous system.

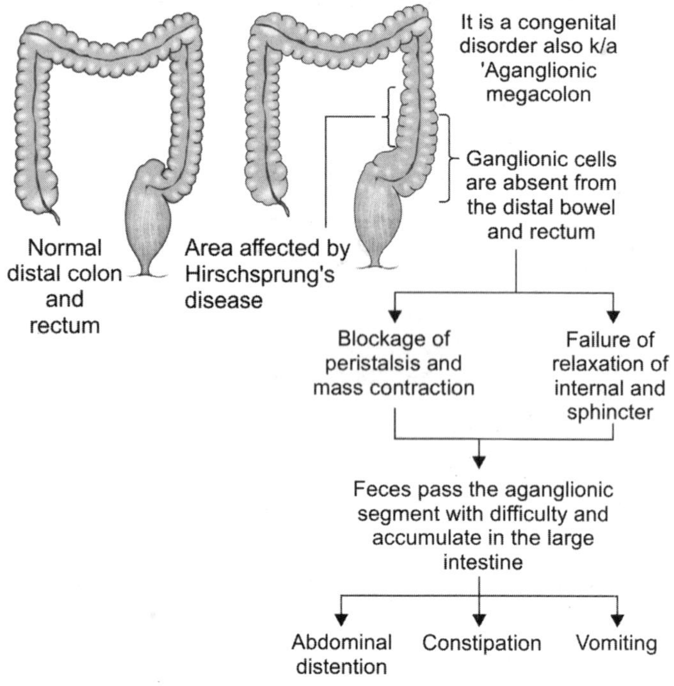

Fig. 3.7: Pathophysiology of Hirschsprung's disease.

4 CHAPTER Cardiovascular Physiology

PY 5.6 Describe abnormal ECG, arrhythmias, heart block and myocardial infarction.
PY 5.11 Describe the pathophysiology of shock, syncope and heart failure.

LEARNING OBJECTIVES

After finishing this module, you should be able to:
- Analyze the clinical problem on the basis of its signs and symptoms, laboratory findings, to reach a differential diagnosis for that problem.
- Describe the pathophysiology of the given clinical condition based on the clinical and laboratory findings.
- Discuss the rationale of management, based on the derangement of physiological parameters in a case scenario.

CASE 4.1 HEART BLOCK

History: A 55 year-old female presents to the emergency department with complaints of lightheadedness, dizziness and syncope. She states that she is having trouble climbing the stairs at home. On leading questions she denies chest pain, cough or other symptoms

She is a known case of hypertension since last 10 years on treatment and Type 2 DM taking oral hypoglycemic agent with history of ischemic heart disease.

- **On examination:** Vital signs are normal except for a pulse of 50 bpm.
- **GPE:** No signs of anemia, jaundice, clubbing, edema and lymphadenopathy
- **Vitals:** Temp–N, BP–130/86 mm of Hg, Pulse rate–50/min
- **RS exam:** No significant abnormal findings
- **CVS exam:** No significant abnormal findings except for bradycardia
- **Investigations:**
  - *ECG:* Sinus Bradycardia and prolonged PR interval.

Based on the above clinical scenario answer the following questions:
1. What is your probable diagnosis?
2. What is the physiological basis of the PR interval?
3. What does a Prolonged PR interval indicate?
4. Name one physiological condition of sinus bradycardia and explain its physiological basis?

Provisional diagnosis: *Atrioventricular conduction block*
- Heart block is a common finding in patients of ischemic heart disease.
- Disturbance in the normal transmission of impulses generated by the SA node results in varying degrees of heart block. There are three types of heart block.
- Most common type of heart block seen in clinical practice is the AV nodal block:

There are three types of heart block or AV nodal blocks:

1. **First degree heart block:** When the electrical signals are slow to reach the ventricles it is known as First degree heart block characterized by consistent prolonged PR interval in the ECG. However all the signals eventually reach the ventricles. Clinically they are asymptomatic and generally do not require any treatment.

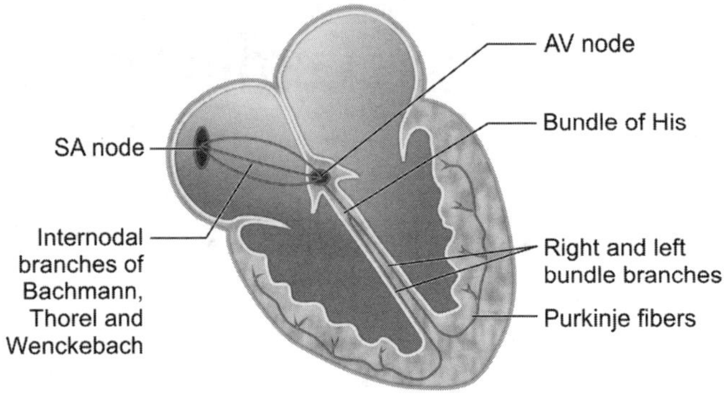

Fig. 4.1: Conducting system of heart showing the transmission of impulse from SA node to cardiac muscle.

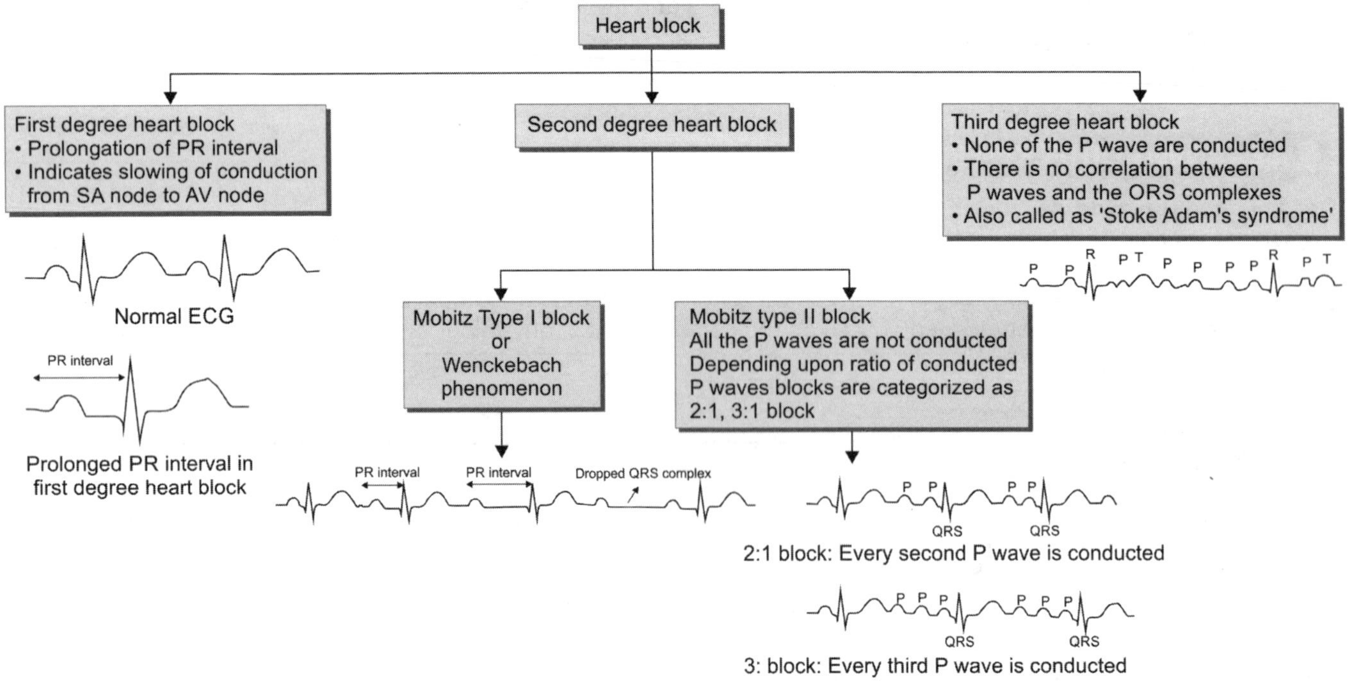

Fig. 4.2: Classification of heart blocks.

2. **Second degree heart block:**
   a. *Type I:* Also known as Wenckebach block or Mobitz Type I AV block. There is increased delay in the conduction of the signals with each heart beat until a beat is missed completely.
   ECG: Progressive prolongation of PR interval followed by P wave without a QRS complex known as blocked P-wave or dropped QRS complex.
   b. *Type II:* Also known as Mobitz type II AV block Some of the electrical signals do not reach the ventricles. It is further categorized as 2:1, 3:1 block.
3. **Third degree heart block:**
   - Also known as complete heart block ***'Stokes-Adams syndrome'.***
   - There is a defect in the conduction system of the heart due to which there is no conduction through the atrioventricular node (AVN) resulting in complete disassociation between the atria and the ventricles. The ventricular escape mechanism can occur anywhere from the AVN to the bundle-branch Purkinje system.

CASE 4.2 WOLFF-PARKINSON-WHITE (WPW) SYNDROME

A 16-years-old adolescent male complained of palpitations and syncope after running on the treadmill for 20 minutes. There is a similar history of palpitations in the past few months. The physical examination shows no significant abnormal findings, however there is tachycardia present. ECG shows supraventricular tachycardia, with shortened PR intervals along with broad QRS complexes and the presence of delta waves (slurring of upstroke of QRS complex).

Based on the above case scenario answer the following questions:
1. What is your probable diagnosis?
2. Support your findings from the history and investigations.
3. What is the pathophysiology behind this disease?
4. What is the cause for the appearance of delta waves in the QRS complex?

Provisional diagnosis: Wolff-Parkinson-White (WPW) syndrome.

WPW syndrome is a congenital disorder characterized by the presence of additional aberrant nodal tissue connection between atria and ventricles (called as bundle of Kent). This conducts more rapidly than AV nodes and one ventricle is excited early.

There are supraventricular tachyarrhythmias present with episodes of palpitation and syncope, which gets precipitated on exertion.

ECG findings: Short PR interval, prolonged QRS complex with delta waves (slurring of upstroke of QRS complexes). This ***'Delta wave'*** occurs because the action potential from the sinoatrial node is able to conduct to the ventricles very quickly through the accessory pathway, and thus the QRS occurs immediately after the P wave.

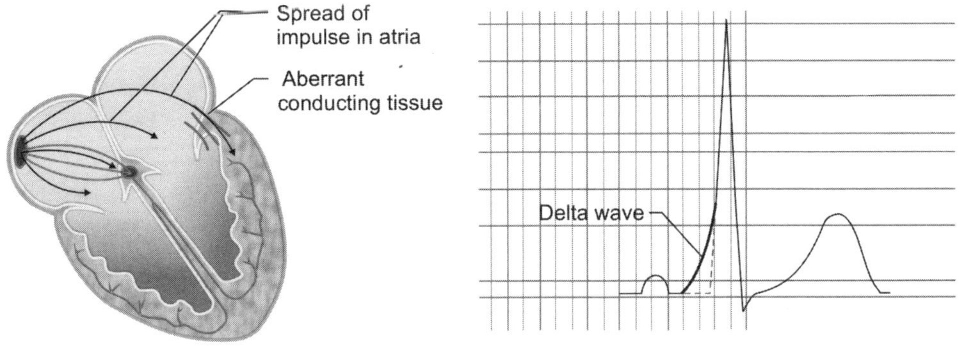

Fig. 4.3: Aberrant conducting tissue (bundle of Kent) and ECG changes in WPW syndrome.

CASE 4.3 CARDIAC FAILURE

History: A 55-year-old male presents to OPD with complaints of shortness of breath. This breathlessness is associated with normal exertion which, a few years back, he could do without any problem. During sleep, he often gets an attack of severe shortness of breath and coughing which awakes him from sleep. This episode of coughing persists even in sitting position.

General physical examination: The patient is calm, conscious, well oriented to time, place and person. Pulse-90/min with characteristic pulsus alternans, BP = 130/90 mm Hg, pitting edema is seen on the ankles (++), jugular venous pressure (JVP) is 4 cm.

Systemic examination of:
- **Abdomen** shows hepatomegaly.
- **Respiratory system:** Bilateral dull percussion note on costophrenic angles.
- **Auscultation** reveals the basal crepitations in both the lungs.
- **Cardiovascular system:**
  - X Ray chest: Cardiomegaly.
  - ECG shows signs of right and left ventricular hypertrophy.
  - 2D echocardiography shows dilation of all the cardiac chambers with poor contractility of cardiac walls and reduced ejection fraction.

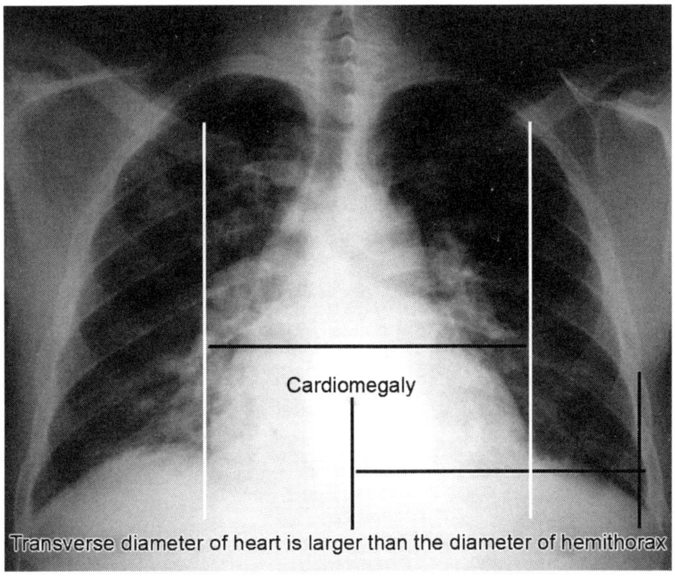

Figure 4.4: PA view of chest.

Based on above clinical condition, answer the following questions:

1. What is the cause of shortness of breath in this patient?
2. What is the cause of increased pulse rate in this patient?
3. What is the cause of raised JVP and liver enlargement in this patient?
4. What is the cause of bilateral dull percussion notes in the chest?
5. What is the cause of basal crepitations in the chest?
6. What is your probable diagnosis based on physical and lab findings?
7. How can you manage this patient keeping in view the pathophysiology of this condition?

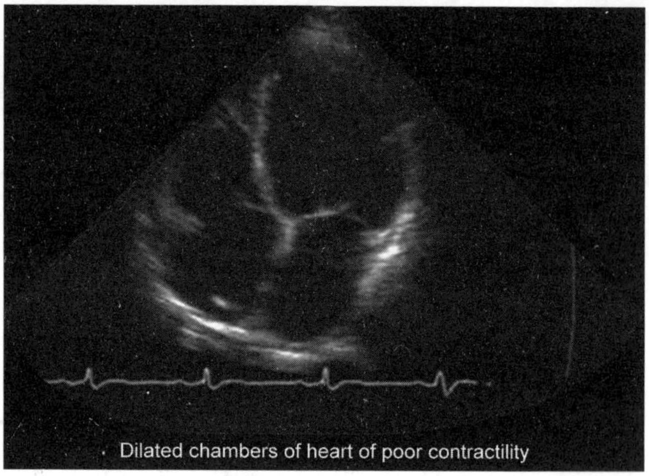

Fig. 4.5: 2-D echocardiography.

Provisional diagnosis: Congestive cardiac failure/biventricular failure.

Cardiac failure is defined as failure of the heart to pump enough blood to meet the demands of the body.

Causes:

- Intrinsic pump failure—weakening of ventricular muscle
- Increased workload on heart, resulting in increased afterload and preload
- Restricted filling of cardiac chambers—cardiac tamponade, constrictive pericarditis.

Depending upon Ventricular Involvement

Single ventricular failure

- **LHF:** Inability of LV to pump the blood into aorta (accumulation of fluid in lungs and pulmonary congestion).
  - *Signs:* Pulmonary edema, pulmonary crepitations present, dyspnea, orthopnea, decreased LV output, ischemic acute tubular necrosis (ATN), hypoxic encephalopathy, muscular weakness and fatigue.
- **RHF (cor pulmonale):** Inability of RV to pump the blood into pulmonary artery.
  - *Signs:* Raised JVP, liver congestion and pedal edema.
- **Biventricular failure:**
  - *Congestive cardiac failure (CCF):* Signs of both LVF and RVF are present.

Pathophysiology of CCF

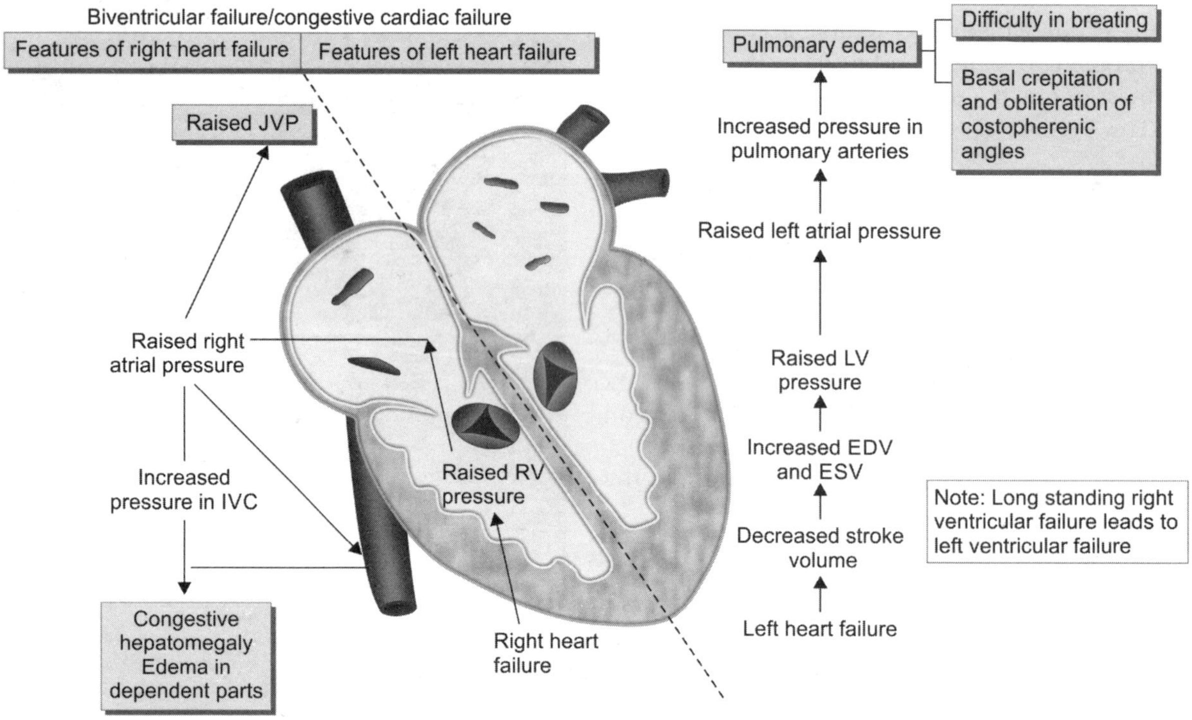

Fig. 4.6: Pathophysiology of congestive cardiac failure.

Physiology of Management of CCF

- **Investigate and diagnose the patient through:**
  - *Chest X-ray:* Shows enlarged shadow of cardiac silhouette.
  - *ECG:* Changes of RVH/LVH or both.
  - *Echocardiography:* Shows CO, valvular movement and ventricular wall thickness and movement.
- **Treatment:**
  - Basic life support
  - Airway maintenance
  - *Oxygen therapy:* To increase the amount of dissolved oxygen resulting in improved tissue oxygenation.
  - *Complete bed rest:* To prevent exertion of heart.
  - *Emotional rest:* To avoid cardiac stress due to catecholamines.
  - *Diet:* Salt and fluid restriction: to reduce volume overload in the body.
  - Drugs:

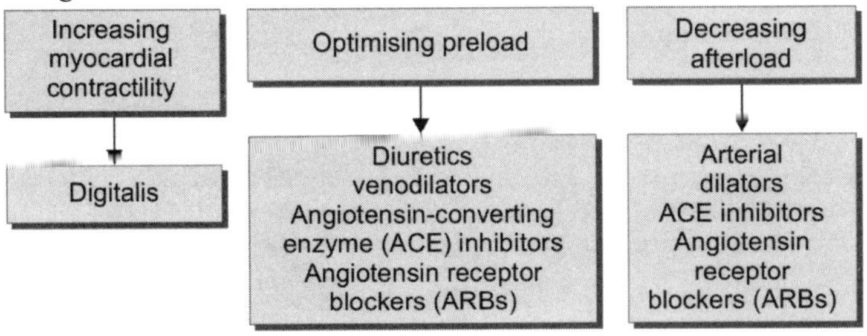

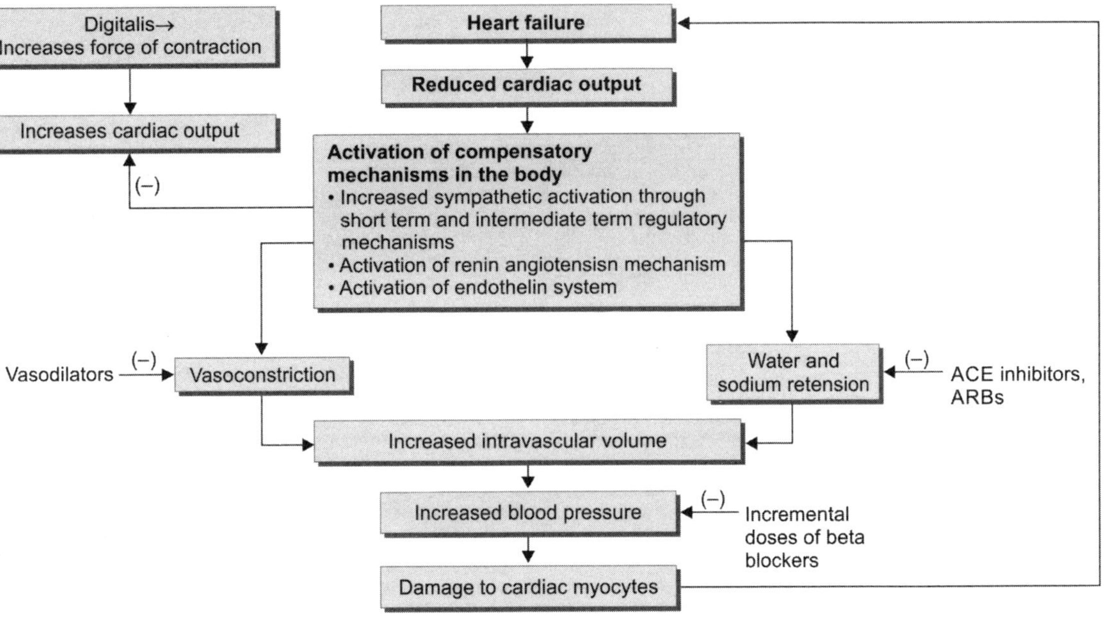

Fig. 4.7: Rationale of drugs in management of CCF.

CASE 4.4 HYPOVOLEMIC SHOCK

History: Parents of a 5-year-old girl had brought her to emergency in a semi-conscious state. She had 7-8 episodes of loose motions and 4 episodes of vomiting in a day. It was associated with intermittent abdomen pain. Previously she had some food from a street vendor.

General physical examination: The patient is drowsy, opening eyes only for painful stimuli. Pulse = 100/min, regular, low volume pulse, BP = 90/70 mm Hg, temperature 100°F. Skin turgor is reduced; mouth and tongue are dry. Respiratory rate is 24/min and shallow.

Based on above clinical condition, answer the following questions:

1. What is your likely diagnosis for this patient?
2. What is the patho-physiology behind this clinical condition?
3. How can you manage this patient based on pathophysiology?

Provisional diagnosis: Severe dehydration due to gastroenteritis resulting in hypovolemic shock.

Shock is a state of inadequate perfusion of the tissues by oxygenated blood and inability of the tissues to utilize the oxygen in the blood.

Causes of Hypovolemic Shock

- Loss of 15–40% of blood volume is fully compensated
- Loss of >40% of blood volume leads to progressive shock

Table 4.1: Causes of hypovolemic shock.

Hemorrhage (most common)	*Loss of plasma volume*	*Loss of body fluids*	*Increased water loss from kidneys*
Surgery Internal bleeding Trauma	Burns	Severe vomiting Severe diarrhea	Diuretics Diabetes insipidus

Stages of Shock

Table 4.2: Stages of shock.

	Stage I	*Stage II*	*Stage III*
Pathogenesis	• Compensatory shock • Compensatory mechanisms come into play	• Progressive shock • Decreased tissue perfusion	• Irreversible shock • Microcirculatory failure • Cellular death • Depletion of ATP
Outcome	• BP normal • Tissue perfusion • Normal	• BP falls • Systemic effects of shock present	Death is imminent

Pathogenesis

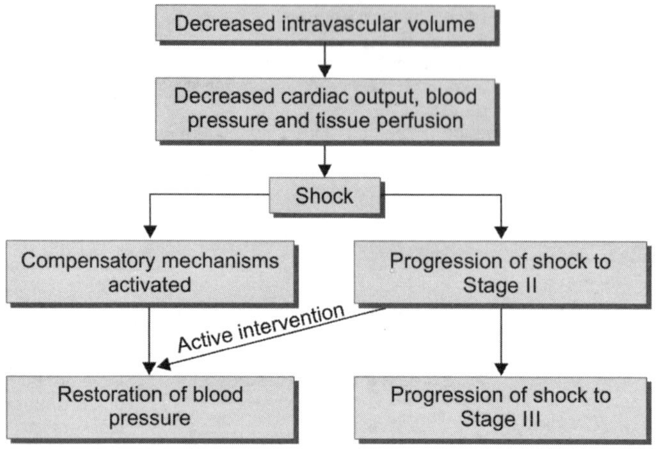

Fig. 4.8: Pathophysiology of hypovolemic shock.

Physiology of Management of Shock

- **Oxygen therapy:** The availability of oxygen will correct the hypoxia and improve the oxygenation of tissues by increasing the levels of dissolved oxygen.
- **Replenish fluid volume:** It is very important in hypovolemic shock.

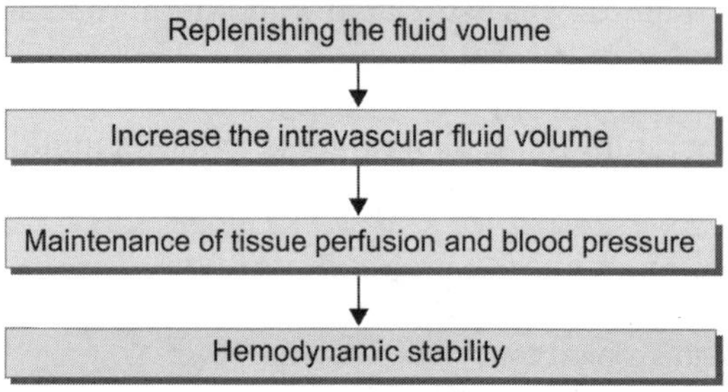

Fig. 4.9: Management of hypovolemic shock.

- Clinical monitoring of vitals
- Glucocorticoids
- Prevent hypothermia.

CASE 4.5 MYOCARDIAL INFARCTION

History: A 68-year-old obese male patient was brought to emergency by ambulance. He complained of sharp, stabbing pain in the center of the chest and discomfort in the left shoulder. He had a previous history of episodes of chest discomfort which he described as chest heaviness. Moderate to heavy exertion were the aggravating factors. He had mild dyspnea and nausea accompanying the pain. He also had intermittent palpitations since last evening.

Physical examination: Vital signs on arrival to the emergency showed a BP of 160/100 mm Hg, pulse = 96/min, and a respiratory rate of 18 per minute. His physical examination did not reveal any other significant finding.

Laboratory Investigations

- Elevated level of enzyme CK-MB
- Elevated level of Troponin -T
- ECG—shows the normal sinus rhythm with ST segment elevation

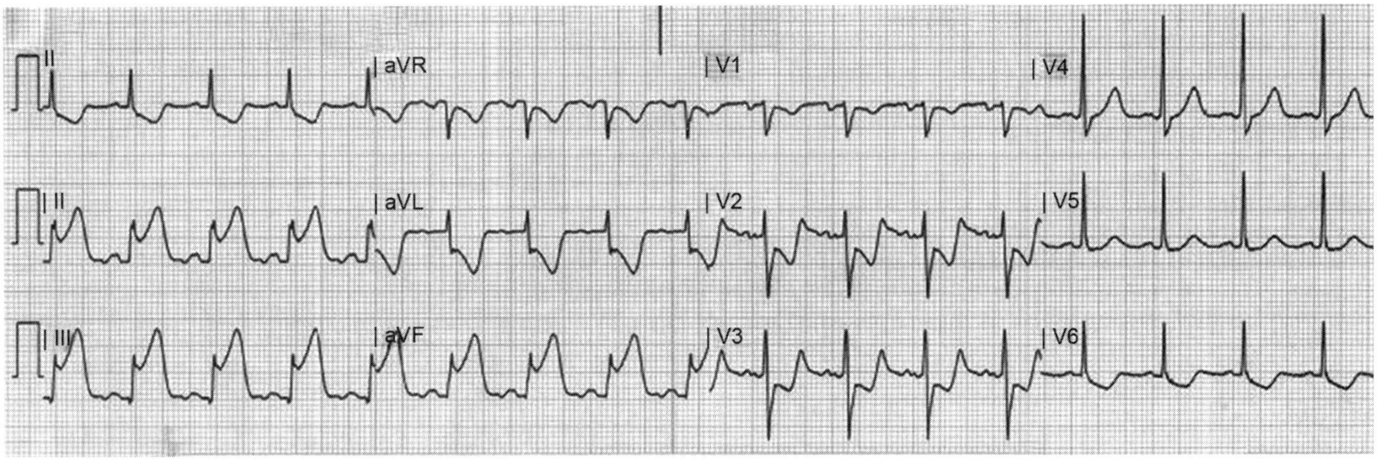

Fig. 4.10: ECG finding of the patient.

- 2D echocardiography shows inferior wall infarct.

Based on above clinical condition, answer the following questions:
1. What is your likely diagnosis for this patient?
2. What is the pathophysiology behind this clinical condition?
3. How can you manage this patient based on pathophysiology?
4. What are the peculiarities of coronary circulation?

Provisional diagnosis: Acute myocardial infarction (inferior wall infarction).
It is the syndrome of ischemia leading to disruption of function and myocardial damage.

Risk Factors

- Males
- Atherosclerosis
- Hyperlipoproteinemia
- Cigarette smoking
- Hypertension
- Diabetes mellitus
- Genetic predisposition

Clinical Presentation

- **Pain:** Deep, visceral, radiating to arm, abdomen, back, lower jaw and neck.
- **Other features:**
  - Weakness
  - Sweating
  - Nausea, vomiting
  - Anxiety
  - Sense of impending doom

Physical Findings

- Patient is pale, anxious, restless, sweating with cold extremities
- Substernal chest pain
- Pulse rate and BP are normal within first hour
- Decreased carotid pulse volume
- Decreased systolic BP

Lab Diagnosis

- **ECG:**
  - ST wave elevation
  - T wave inversion
- **Serum cardiac markers:**
  - CPK-MB
  - Cardiac specific troponin–T
- **Cardiac imaging:**
  - 2-D echocardiography
- **Radionucleotide study:**
  - To study the regional blood flow in heart
  - Thallium (^{201}Tl) is used shows areas of ischemia show low Tl uptake
  - Technetium-99 m is selectively taken up by infarcted area
  - ^{133}Xe washout method combined with angiography to outline the distribution of blood.

Management

- O_2 inhalation
- Inj. Morphine to control pain
- Inj. streptokinase within 6 hours: To clear out the thromboembolic blockage/dissolution of clot
- Low molecular weight heparin: To prevent intravascular clotting
- Low dose aspirin (acts as antiplatelet aggregation drug)
- Surgical treatment:
  - Percutaneous transluminal coronary angioplasty
  - Coronary artery bypass grafting (CABG)

Complications

- **Arrhythmias:**
  - *Dangerous periods:*
    - First 30 minutes
    - 12 hours after MI
    - 3 days to several weeks after MI
- Decreased cardiac output due to **systolic stretch**
- Damming of blood in venous system
- Rupture of infarcted area in cardiac tamponade and sudden death.

5 CHAPTER

Respiratory Physiology

PY 6.5 Describe and discuss the principles of artificial respiration, oxygen therapy, acclimatization and decompression sickness.

LEARNING OBJECTIVES

After finishing this module, you should be able to:

- Analyze the clinical problem on the basis of its signs and symptoms, laboratory findings, to reach a differential diagnosis for that problem.
- Describe the pathophysiology of the given clinical condition based on the clinical and laboratory findings.
- Discuss the rationale of management, based on the derangement of physiological parameters in a case scenario.

CASE 5.1 CAISSON'S DISEASE

History: A 60-year-old Hindu male patient came to our OPD with complaint of breathlessness for the last 5 years and coughing with sputum production for the last 5 years. He was a chronic smoker for the last 30 years. He was symptomatic for most of the months but symptoms used to increase during winter. Initially, he was breathless during doing heavy work only but now he feels breathlessness even while doing routine work also. His sputum was white coloured, purulent in consistency, about 100 mL/day.

General physical examination: He was having tachypnea and tachycardia. His BP was normal but JVP was raised and liver was palpable about 1 cm below right costal margin.

Examination of respiratory system: Revealed bilateral hyperinflated chest with widened intercostal spaces and hyperresonant note on percussion. Chest auscultation revealed bilateral wheezes scattered all over our lung field.

Chest X-ray: Showing bilateral low placed diaphragm with tubular heart.

Routine blood investigations: Were in normal range.

Spirometry: Results showed mild obstructive pattern (FEV_1/FVC ratio <0.61) with no significant reversibility in FEV_1.

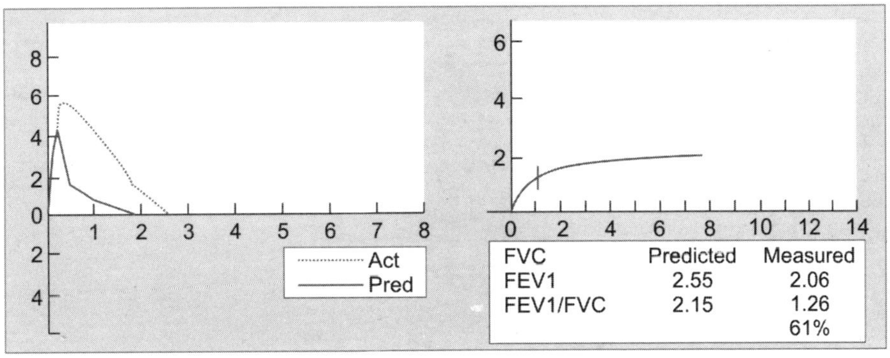

Fig. 5.1: Flow volume loop and timed vital capacity, as seen on spirometry.

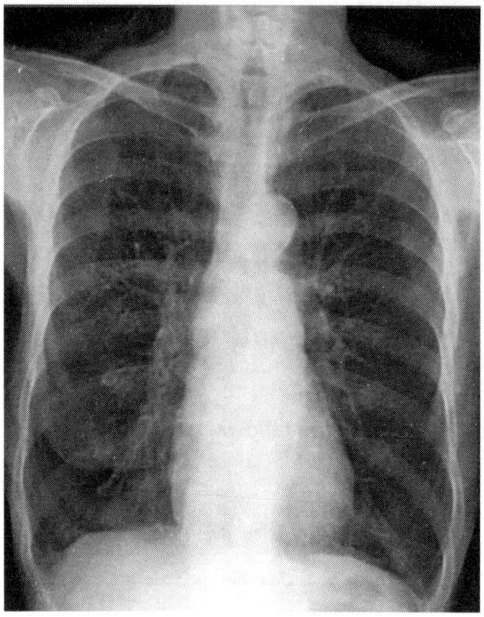

Fig. 5.2: X-ray chest (PA view).

Based on the above case, answer the following questions:

1. What is your provisional diagnosis?
2. What is the cause of breathlessness in this patient?
3. What is the cause of increased respiratory rate in this patient?
4. What is the cause of raised jugular venous pressure and liver enlargement in this patient?
5. What is the cause of hyperresonant percussion note in this patient?
6. What is the cause of expiratory wheeze in this patient?
7. What is the cause of low diaphragm and tubular heart on chest X-ray?
8. What is the significance of FEV_1/FVC ratio?

Provisional diagnosis: Chronic obstructive pulmonary disease (COPD).

Definition: Chronic obstructive pulmonary disease (COPD) is a progressive lung disease characterized by poor reversible airflow obstruction and an abnormal inflammatory response in the lungs.

Pathophysiology of Chronic Obstructive Pulmonary Disease (COPD)

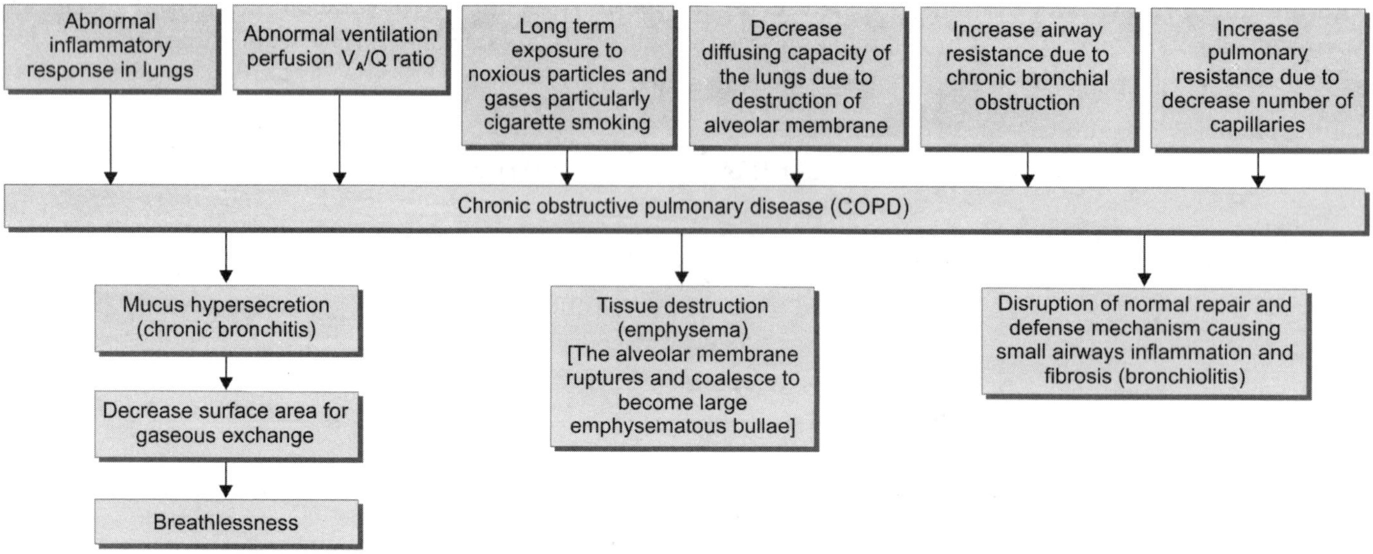

Fig. 5.3: Pathophysiology of COPD.

Physiological basis behind the specific clinical features of chronic obstructive pulmonary disease (COPD)

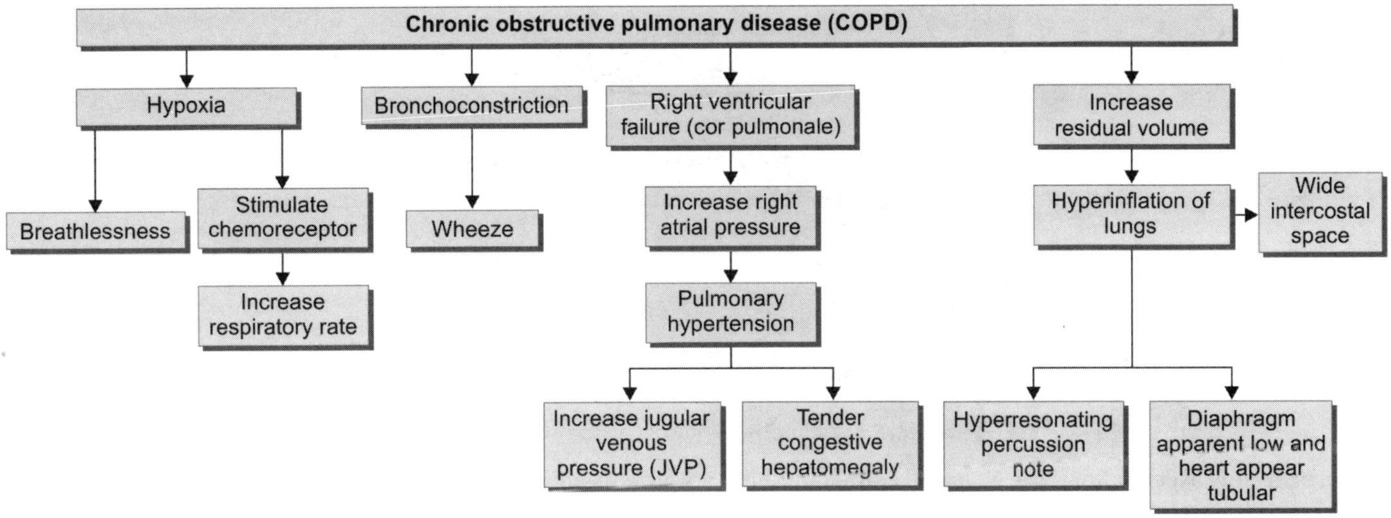

Fig. 5.4: Physiological aspect of clinical features of COPD.

Significance of FEV_1/FVC ratio: It is a very sensitive index to distinguish between obstructive lung disease and restrictive lung disease.

Parameter of spirometer	*Normal*	*Obstructive lung disease*	*Restrictive lung disease*
Forced vital capacity (FVC)	5.0 L	3.0 L	2.5 L
Forced expiratory volume in 1 second (FEV_1)	4.0 L	1.2 L	2.0 L
FEV_1/FVC ratio	80%of FVC	40% of FVC	80% of FVC

CASE 5.2 HIGH ALTITUDE SICKNESS

History: After a 30 minute expedition on the sea bed, the diver was rapidly pulled up by his friends. On resurfacing, he experienced difficulty in breathing, body ache and convulsions.

Clinical examination: Pulse rate—90 pulse per minute. Respiratory rate—16 breaths per minute.

Based on the above case, answer the following questions:
1. What is your provisional diagnosis?
2. What will happen and why if a diver ascends rapidly to the surface after deep dive?
3. What are the physiological basis behind clinical presentation of this disease?
4. What is the depth of sea when person develops nitrogen narcosis?

Provisional diagnosis: Dysbarism/Caisson's disease/Decompression sickness/The bends/Diver's palsy.

Definition

Dysbarism means the effect of pressure difference between the ambient pressure and the pressure of the dissolved and free gases in the body. It is caused due to increased pN_2 in the blood. This clinical condition is found in the person, who was previously surrounded with a high pressure environment and rapidly brought to low pressure surroundings.

Pathophysiology

It happens in deep sea divers, who are subjected to high atmospheric pressure on the ocean bed as compared to sea level atmospheric pressure. The inspired air, at sea level, has 80% N_2 and 20% O_2 mixture, which gets dissolved (esp. N_2) in the adipose tissue of the diver. On a rapid ascent to surface, this N_2 bubbles and block the microvasculature and results in a typical clinical picture, as shown in diagram below:

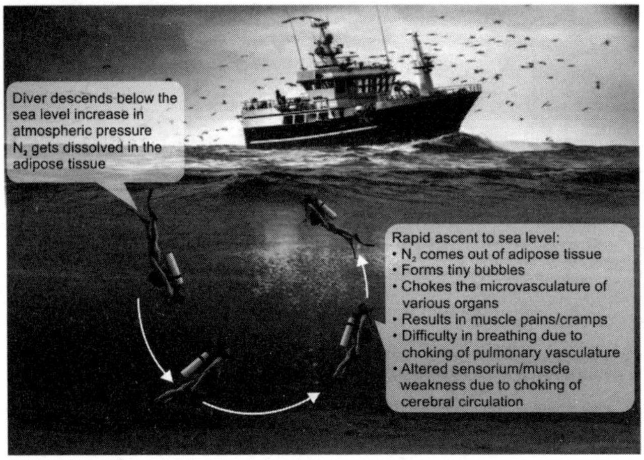
Diver descends below the sea level increase in atmospheric pressure N_2 gets dissolved in the adipose tissue
Rapid ascent to sea level:
• N_2 comes out of adipose tissue
• Forms tiny bubbles
• Chokes the microvasculature of various organs
• Results in muscle pains/cramps
• Difficulty in breathing due to choking of pulmonary vasculature
• Altered sensorium/muscle weakness due to choking of cerebral circulation

Fig. 5.5: Pathophysiology of Caisson's disease.

However, a slow ascent allows the N_2 gas to come out of the adipose tissue and dissolve in blood, resulting in a natural and uneventful elimination from the diver's body.

Management

The diver, when exposed to high pressure, by keeping him in a pressurised chamber, will re-dissolve the bubbles of nitrogen gas in body fluid. Then a slow decompression will allow the nitrogen to un-dissolve in a controlled manner. This liberated nitrogen gets out of the body through lungs. Hyperbaric oxygen therapy is also helpful in recovery.

CASE 5.3 ACUTE MOUNTAIN SICKNESS

History: Satish, 20 year old, resident of Delhi, went for a 4 day trip to a hill station (2900 m height) in Himachal Pradesh. Few hours after reaching the hill station, he started to feel mental and physical fatigue, headache, dizziness and nausea.

Clinical examination:
- Radial pulse rate—76 pulse per minute
- Respiratory rate—17 breaths per minute
- Body temperature— 97°F.

Based on the above case, answer the following questions:
1. What is your provisional diagnosis?
2. What will happen to the ventilation of patient with hypoxic hypoxia?
3. Why does a person develop pulmonary edema at a very high altitude?

Provisional diagnosis: Acute mountain sickness.

Definition: Satish seems to be suffering from acute mountain sickness. He is a resident of Delhi. During the trip to a hill station he was exposed to an environment of low partial oxygen pressure. This environmental condition led to hypoxic hypoxia. Generally, the symptoms of acute mountain sickness begin at an altitude of above 12000 feet. The prominent symptoms include drowsiness, mental and physical fatigue, headache, nausea. The severity of symptoms increases with altitude.

Severe cases may lead to high altitude pulmonary edema and high altitude cerebral edema.

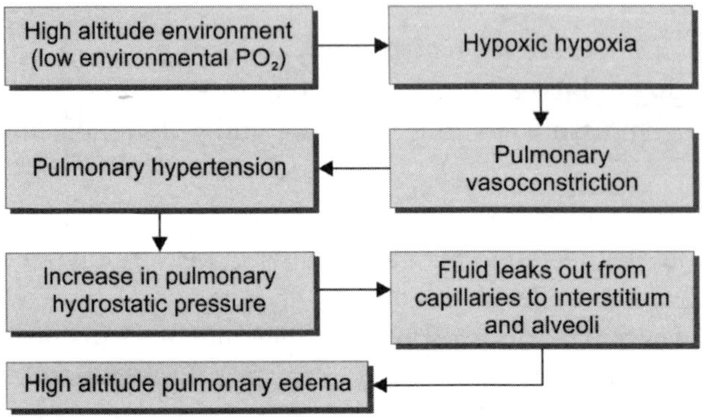

Fig. 5.6: Pathophysiology of acute mountain sickness.

If you compare the above mentioned pathophysiology, then you will be able to point out one interesting response of pulmonary circulation and peripheral circulation for hypoxia. On one hand hypoxia causes vasodilation in peripheral circulation, on the other hand it causes vasoconstriction in pulmonary circulation.

Management

- The best step for managing this condition is bringing the person to a lower altitude.
- **Diuretics:** It acts by reducing the fluid load in the body. Acetazolamide, which is a carbonic anhydrase inhibitor, increases the bicarbonate ion loss in urine. So, by decreasing the alkali load of the body, it helps in maintaining hypoxia as a respiratory drive.
- **Steroids:** It is useful in case of cerebral edema. It acts by decreasing the permeability of the blood brain barrier.
- Hyperbaric oxygen.

6 CHAPTER Renal Physiology

PY 7.6 Describe the innervations of the urinary bladder, physiology of micturition and its abnormalities.
PY 7.7 Describe artificial kidney, dialysis and renal transplantation.

LEARNING OBJECTIVES

After finishing this module, you should be able to:
- Analyze the clinical problem on the basis of its signs and symptoms, laboratory findings, to reach a differential diagnosis for that problem.
- Describe the pathophysiology of the given clinical condition based on the clinical and laboratory findings.
- Discuss the rationale of management, based on the derangement of physiological parameters in a case scenario.

CASE 6.1 NEUROGENIC BLADDER

A 44-year-old male comes to the urologist with pain in the suprapubic region and dribbling micturition. He had met with a Road Traffic Accident (RTA) one year back with complete transaction of the spinal cord at the level of L_{4}-L_{5} and is now in the recovery phase. On leading question, the patient confirms that he has to void urine at regular intervals. Patient is normotensive, non-diabetic, non-smoker and a social drinker.

On Examination

Patient is conscious, co-operative well-oriented to time, place and person.
- Vitals: Normal
- General physical examination (GPE): Normal
- CNS examination: Findings are consistent as in the recovery phase after a spinal injury.

Investigations

- Urine routine examination: Pus cells—40-50/Hpf
- Albumin—trace
- Sugar and ketones—absent

Based on the above case, answer the following questions:
1. What is your provisional diagnosis?
2. Enumerate the various bladder dysfunctions.
3. Describe the innervation of the urinary bladder.

Provisional diagnosis: Neurogenic bladder/Automatic bladder.

Definition: It is defined as dysfunction of the bladder resulting from diseases of the CNS or peripheral nerves that control micturition.

Pathophysiology

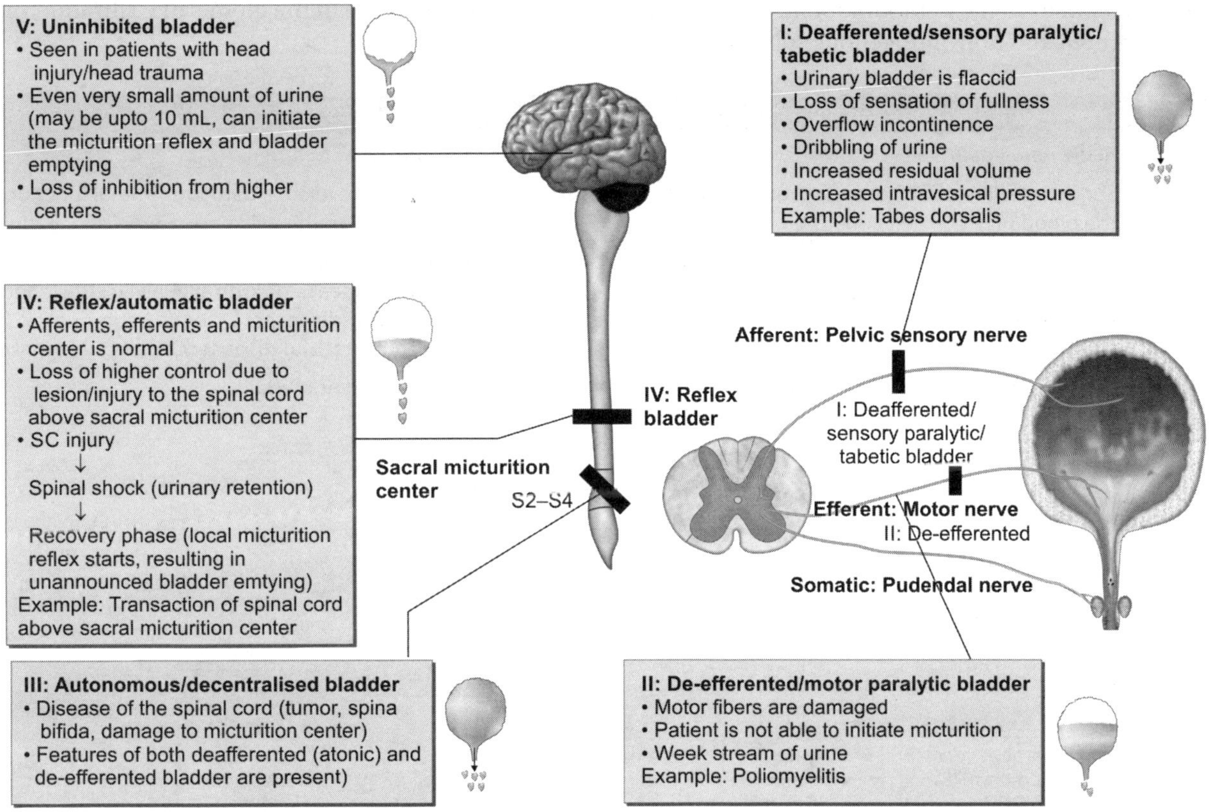

Fig. 6.1: Pathophysiology of neurogenic bladder dysfunction.

CASE 6.2 CHRONIC RENAL FAILURE

A 41-year-old male with a long-standing history of hypertension and diabetes presents with complaints of pruritus, lethargy, lower extremity edema, nausea and emesis. He denies any other medical illness.

On Examination

The patient is well oriented to time, place and person. He is average in built and nourishment with mild respiratory distress.

Blood pressure 180/110 mm of Hg, pulse 80/minute, respiratory rate 24/minute and is afebrile. The patient looks pale, there is mild edema on lower extremities (2+) with superficial excoriations of his skin due to scratching.

Lab Investigations

- **Hb:** 8 g%.
- **Serum creatinine:** 16 mg/dL (reference value <1 mg/dL).
- **Blood urea nitrogen:** 170 mg/dL (reference value 20–40 mg/dL).
- Serum potassium 6.2 mmol/liter (reference value between 3.5 and 5.0 mmol/L).
- Parathormone levels are elevated.

Based on above clinical condition answer the following questions:

1. What is your probable diagnosis? How did you arrive at this conclusion?
2. What would be the physiological basis of the management?
3. Why does the patient have nausea, emesis, lethargy and pruritus?
4. Why is the parathyroid hormone elevated?
5. What according to you could be the role of kidneys in hypertension here?
6. What is the significance of estimating serum creatine and in this patient?
7. What are the systemic manifestations of chronic renal failure?
8. When do you label a patient with end stage renal disease?
9. How can you manage a patient with end-stage renal disease?

Provisional diagnosis: Chronic renal failure .

Renal Failure

Definition: It is defined as the deterioration in renal functions that leads to decrease in the glomerular filtration rate (GFR) with a rise in the urea and non-nitrogenous substances in the blood.

Table 6.1: Differences in acute and chronic renal failure.

	Acute renal failure	*Chronic renal failure*
Onset	Sudden decline of GFR over days or weeks with rapid rise in the blood urea	Slow and irreversible damage of renal functions resulting in uremia
Causes	**Pre-renal:** Severe hemorrhage, shock, burns, hypovolemia, septicemia **Intra-renal:** Acute glomerulonephritis, acute tubular necrosis **Obstructive:** Urinary tract infection	**Congenital:** Polycystic kidney **Vascular disease of kidney:** Polyarteritis nodosa **Glomerular diseases:** Diabetic nephropathy **Tubulointerstitial disease:** Obstructive renal disease
Urine volume	Oliguria and anuria	Polyuria and nocturia

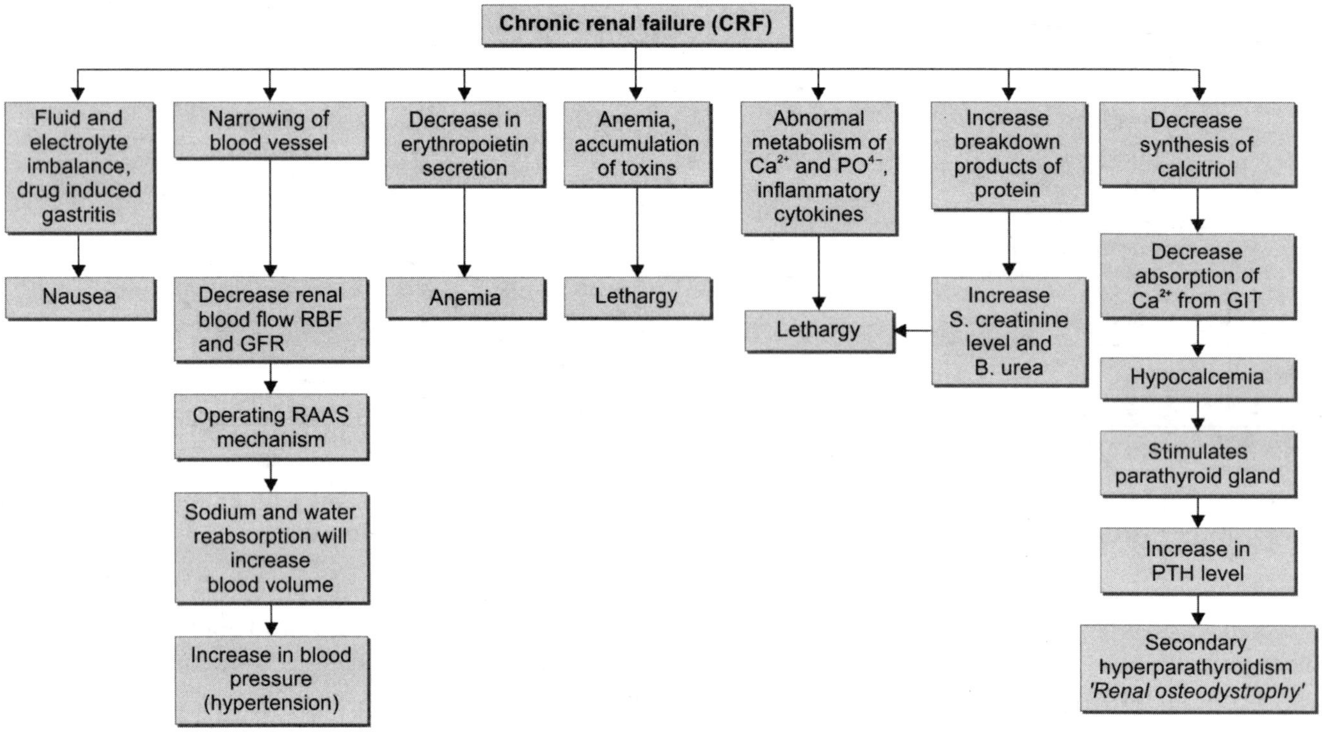

Fig. 6.2: Pathophysiology of chronic renal failure.

Physiology of Management

- Correction of the fluid electrolyte balance
- Salt restricted diet to prevent salt and water overload
- Decrease potassium in the diet to correct hyperkalemia seen in this patient
- Correction of anemia
- Management of hypertension and diabetes mellitus.

7 CHAPTER

Endocrine Physiology

PY 8.2: **Describe the synthesis, secretion, transport, physiological actions, regulation and effect of altered (hypo and hyper) secretion of pituitary gland, thyroid gland, parathyroid gland, adrenal gland, pancreas and hypothalamus.**
PY 8.4: **Describe function tests: Thyroid gland; adrenal cortex, adrenal medulla and pancreas.**

LEARNING OBJECTIVES

After finishing this module, you should be able to:

- Analyze the clinical problem on the basis of its signs and symptoms, laboratory findings, to reach a differential diagnosis for that problem.
- Describe the pathophysiology of the given clinical condition based on the clinical and laboratory findings.
- Discuss the rationale of management, based on the derangement of physiological parameters in a case scenario.

CASE 7.1 HYPOTHYROIDISM

History: A 50-year-old housewife complains of progressive weight gain of 5 kg in 1 year, fatigue, slight memory loss, slow speech, dry skin, constipation, and cold intolerance.

Physical examination: Vital signs include a temperature 96.8°F, pulse 58/minute and regular, BP 140/100 mm Hg. She is moderately obese and speaks slowly and has a puffy face, with pale, cool, dry, and thick skin. The thyroid gland is slightly enlarged, firm, not nodular, mobile, and not tender. The deep tendon reflex time is delayed.

Lab investigations:

- CBC and differential WBC are normal.
- Serum T4 concentration is 3.8 ug/dL (Reference value: 5–12 μg/dL)
- Serum TSH is 23.0 mIU/L (Reference value: 0.4–4.0 mIU/L)
- Serum cholesterol is 255 mg/dL (Reference value: <240 mg/dL)

Based on the above clinical scenario answer the following questions:

1. What is your probable diagnosis?
2. What is the physiological basis of elevated TSH level?
3. What is the physiological basis of clinical features of this disease?
4. Describe the synthesis of thyroid hormone.

Provisional diagnosis: Primary hypothyroidism.

Primary hypothyroidism: When hypothyroidism develop due to the disease or causes that primarily affect thyroid gland.

Causes:

- Auto-immune thyroiditis (Hashimoto's thyroiditis)
- Iatrogenic (postsurgical, radioiodine ^{131}I exposure)
- Drugs (lithium, excess use of antithyroid drugs)
- Congenital disorders (inborn errors of thyroid synthesis, abnormal thyroid gland)
- Iodine deficiency

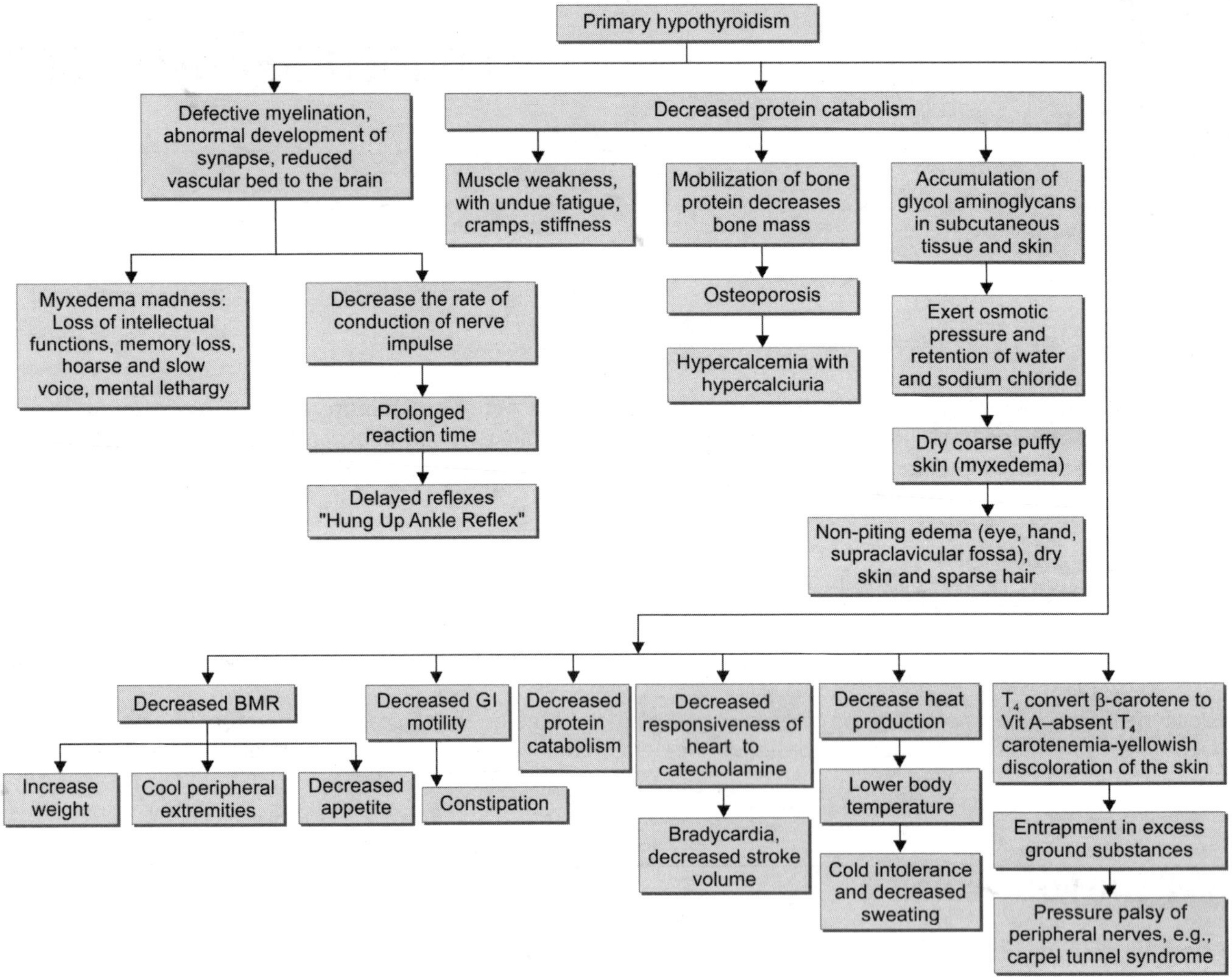

Fig. 7.1: Physiological basis of clinical feature of primary hypothyroidism.

Regulation of thyroid hormone secretion: Increased level of TSH in primary hypothyroidism is due to decreased negative feedback mechanism.

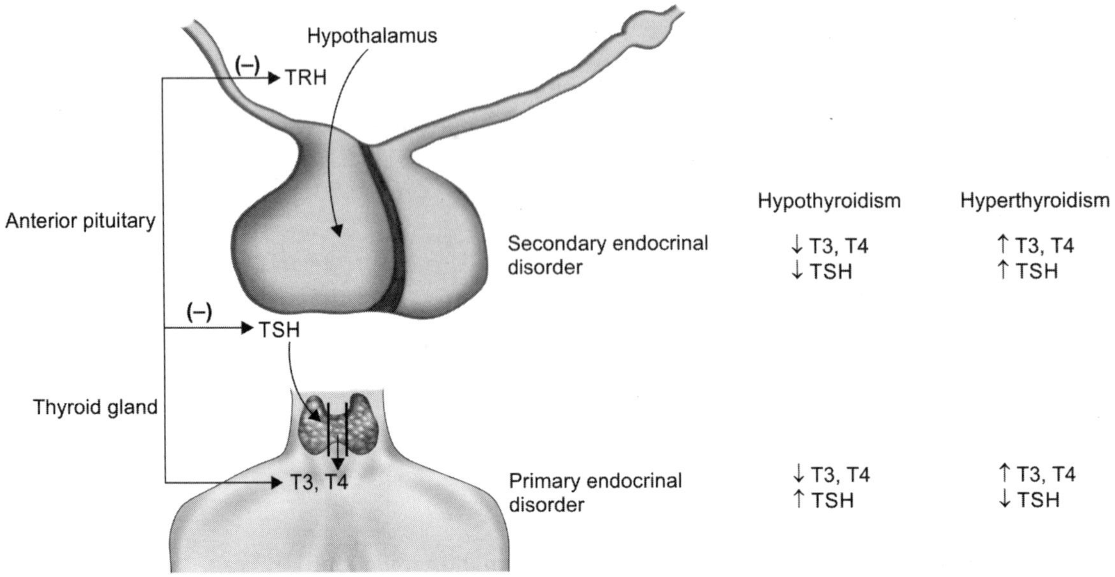

Fig. 7.2: Regulation of throid hormone secretion.

CASE 7.2 HYPERTHYROIDISM

A 35-year-old nurse complained of nervousness, mood swings, weakness, and palpitations with exertion for the past 6 months. Recently, she noticed excessive sweating and wanted to sleep with fewer blankets than her husband. Menstrual periods had been regular but there was less bleeding.

Physical examination: Pulse was 92/minute and BP was 130/60 mm Hg. She appeared anxious, with a smooth, warm, and moist skin, a fine tremor, a bounding cardiac apical impulse, a pulmonic flow murmur, and her thyroid was not palpable and there was no lymphadenopathy. Her eyes were not prominent (proptotic) and she had no focal skin thickening.

Lab Investigations

- Serum T4 = 20.6 µg/dL (Reference value: 5–12 µg/dL)
- Serum T3 = 3.0 µg/dL (Reference value: 5.0–12.0 µg/dL)
- Serum TSH is 0.15 IU/mL (Reference value: 0.4–3.5 IU/mL)

Based on the above clinical scenario answer the following questions:

1. What is your probable diagnosis?
2. What is the physiological basis of decreased TSH level?
3. What is the physiological basis of warm and moist skin?

Provisional Diagnosis

Primary Hyperthyroidism

It is the condition resulting from increased circulating levels of T_4 and T_3. The most common cause is Grave's disease (exophthalmic goiter) or thyrotoxicosis. It is an autoimmune disorder.

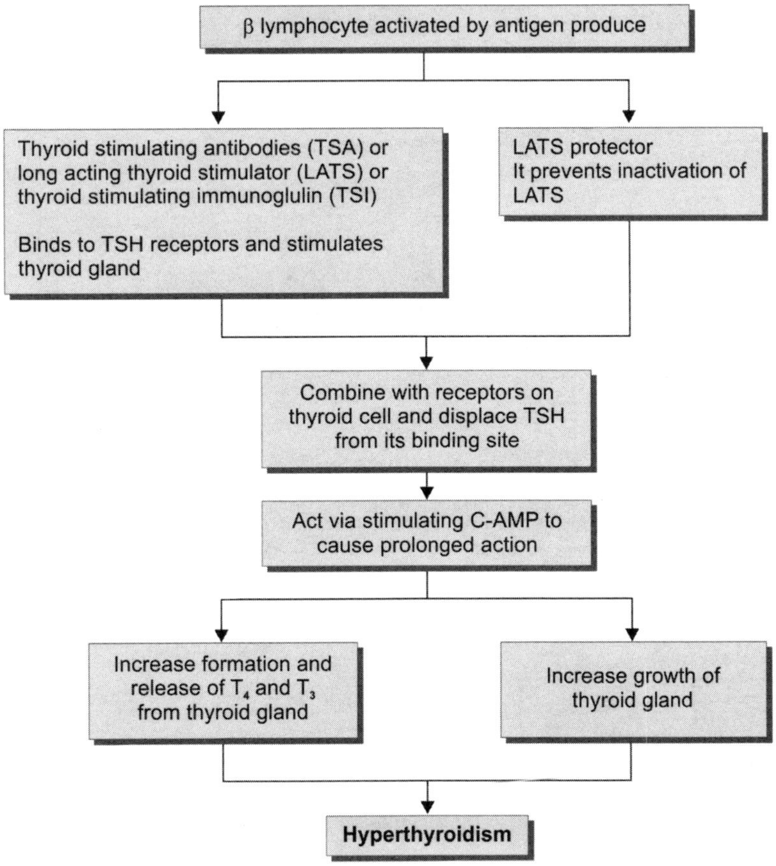

Fig. 7.3: Pathophysiology of hyperthyroidism.

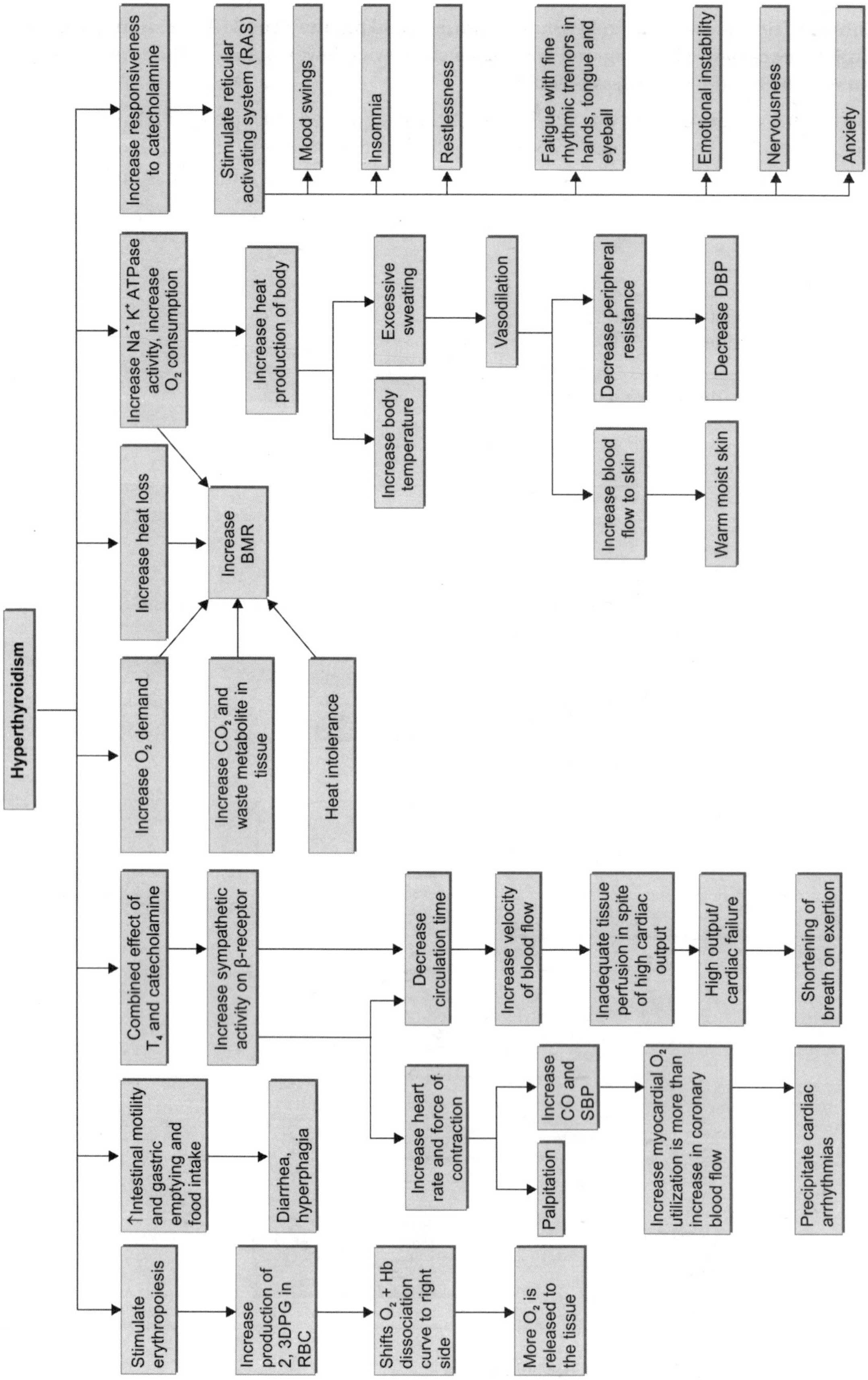

Fig. 7.4A: Physiological basis of clinical features of hyperthyroidism.

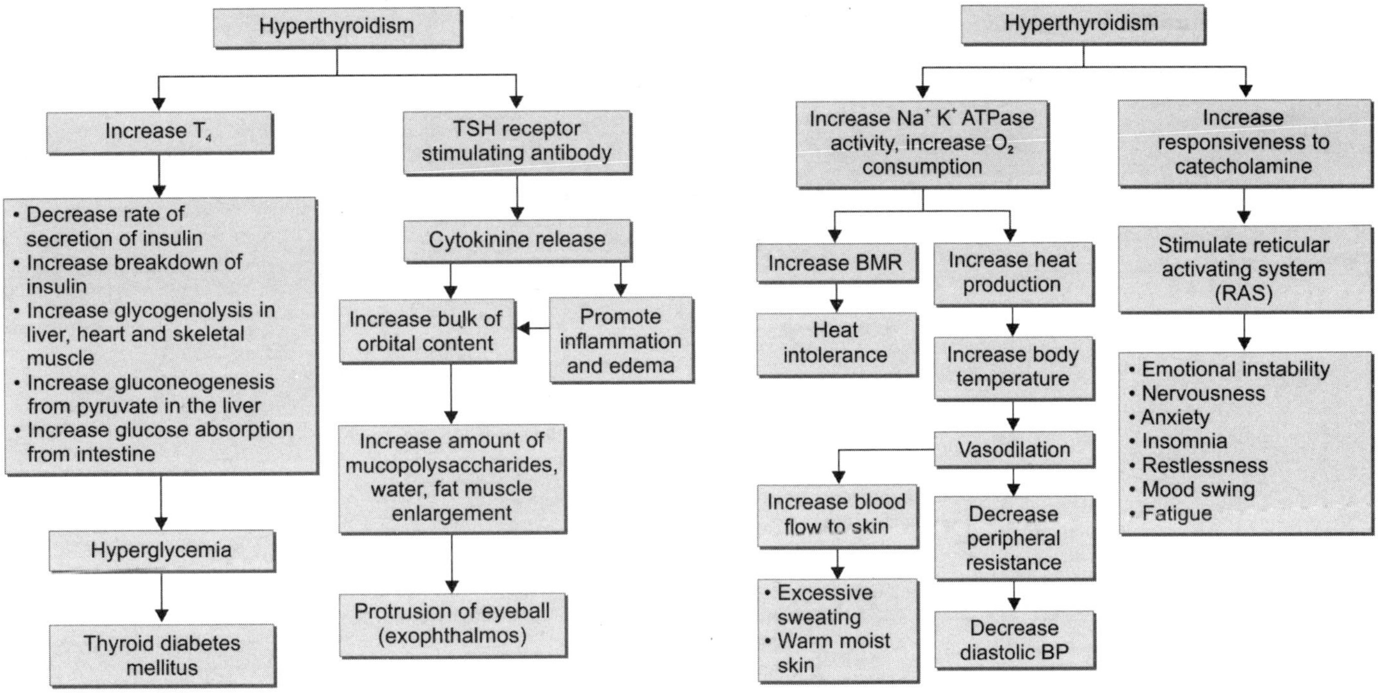

Fig. 7.4B: Physiological basis of clinical features of hyperthyroidism.

CASE 7.3 ACROMEGALY

History: A 35-year-old woman presents with a history of acne, oily skin, and mild hirsutism with elevated testosterone levels. The patient also complains of excessive sweating and some gradual enlargement of her hands and feet, such that she recently had to resize a ring that she has worn for years. Her menstrual cycles have become more irregular. Upon further questioning, she states that she has started to snore and occasionally has a headache upon awakening. The patient has also noticed some disturbance with the vision.

Physical examination: The patient is calm, conscious, well oriented to time, place and person.

Pulse = 80/min

BP = 120/80 mm Hg

She has a protruding jaw with an enlarged tongue. There is significant soft tissue thickening, enlargement of the hands and feet and kyphosis. There is mild facial hirsutism; no acanthosis nigricans. Perimetry show bitemporal hemianopia. Rest of the examination revealed no significant findings.

Laboratory Findings

- Random growth hormone levels of 19.3 ng/mL (reference value: <2.5 ng/mL).
- IGF-I: 910 ng/mL (reference value: 115–307 ng/mL)
- Serum prolactin was within normal range.
- Fasting blood glucose levels: 140 mg/dL (reference value: <110 mg/dL)
- MRI scan of head reveals pituitary adenoma pressing upon the optic chiasma.

Based on the above clinical scenario answer the following questions:

1. What is your probable diagnosis?
2. What is the pathophysiology of this disease?
3. What is the physiological basis of elevated fasting blood sugar?
4. What is the physiological basis the visual disturbance?

Provisional diagnosis: Acromegaly.

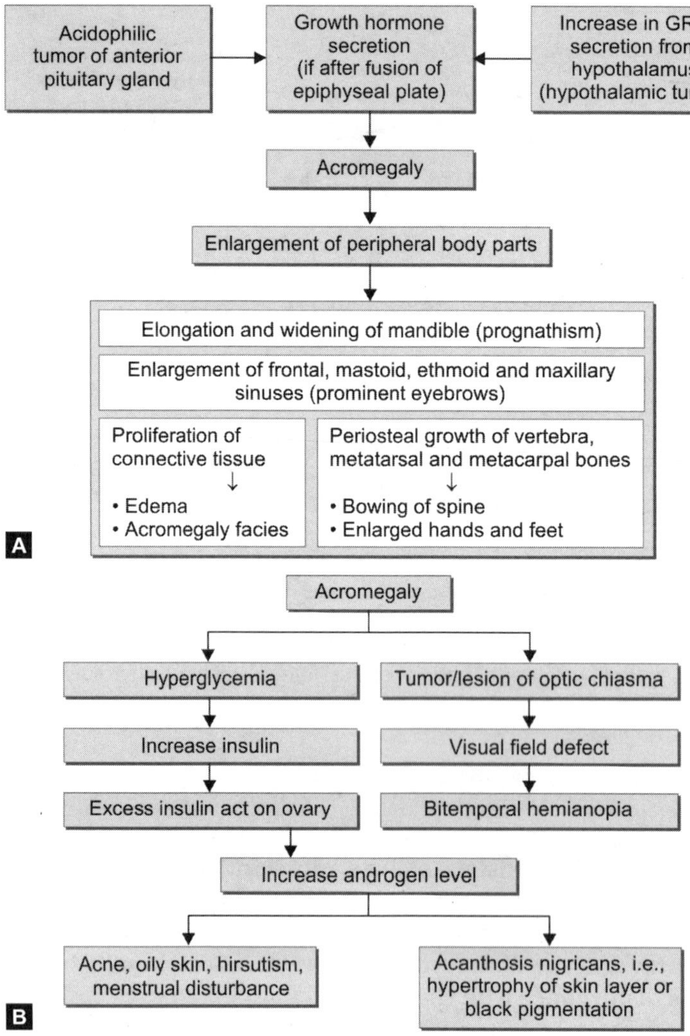

Figs. 7.5A and B: Physiological basis of clinical features of acromegaly.

CASE 7.4 CUSHING'S SYNDROME

History: A 27-year-old female presented with a complaint of gain in weight of approximately 10 kg over 1 year. She also complained of increased blood loss during her periods. There has been an increase in acne and growth of facial hair on chin and upper lips. She said that she feels depressed and unhappy due to her present condition. Recently she had a constant pain in her back with difficulty in walking.

Physical examination:
- The patient is calm, conscious, well oriented to time, place and person. Pulse = 80/min, BP = 130/90 mm Hg.
- Moon like face and fragile skin.
- There is a collection of subcutaneous fat at the base of her neck (buffalo hump). There is truncal obesity with thin limbs.
- There are pupural striae on the abdominal wall.
- Lower back pain, radiating to legs. Tenderness over L4,5.

Lab Investigations

- **Fasting blood sugar:** 156 mg/dL (Reference value: <100 mg/dL)
- Serum cholesterol: 285 mg/dL (Reference value: <240 mg/dL)
- Triglycerides: 168 mg/dL (Reference value: <1500 mg/dL)
- Cortisol: 39 μg/dL (Reference value—early morning levels: 10–20 μg/dL)
- DHEA (dehydroepiandrosterone): 468 μg/dL (Reference value: 65 to 380μg/dL in 25–30 years old female)

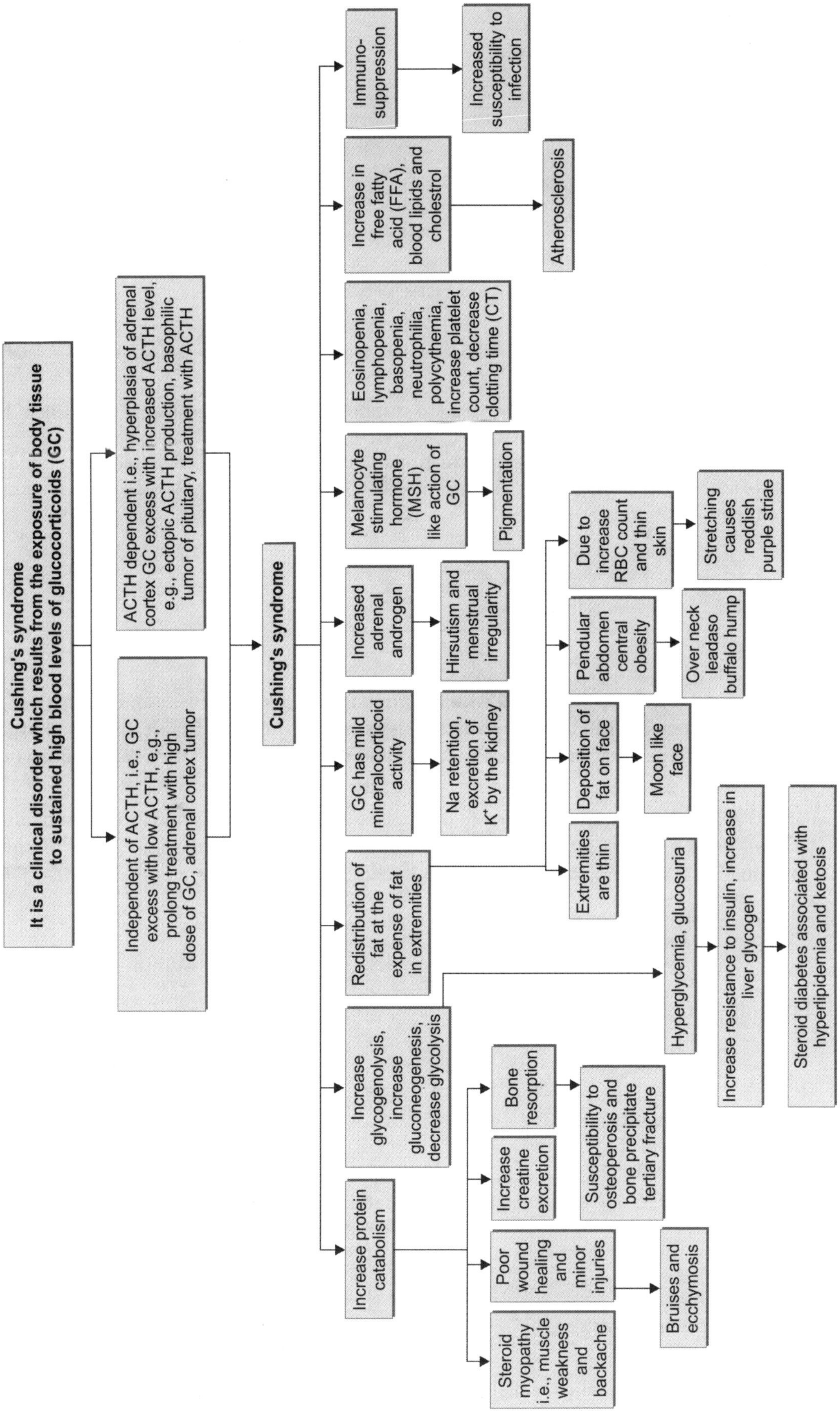

Fig. 7.6: Physiological basis of clinical features of Cushing's syndrome.

- Testosterone: 94 ng/dL (Reference value: 15–70 ng/dL in women)
- ↑ACTH (adrenocorticotropic hormone) raised.
- **X-ray spine:** Compression fracture between L4-L5, osteoporosis.
- **CT scan of abdomen:** A mass seen in the left adrenal gland.

Based on the above clinical scenario answer the following questions:
1. What is your probable diagnosis?
2. What is the pathophysiology of this clinical condition?
3. Explain the physiological basis for:
   A. Increased fasting blood glucose level.
   B. Increase in facial hairs in female patient.
   C. Purple striae on the abdomen wall.
   D. Osteoporosis in these patients.
   E. Delayed wound healing.
   F. Truncal obesity.

Provisional diagnosis: Cushing's syndrome

It is a clinical disorder which results from the exposure of body tissue to sustained high blood levels of glucocorticoids (GC). It is of two types:
1. Independent of ACTH, i.e., GC excess with low ACTH, e.g., prolonged treatment with high dose of GC, adrenal cortex tumor.
2. ACTH dependent, i.e., hyperplasia of adrenal cortex GC excess with increased ACTH level, e.g., ectopic ACTH production, basophilic tumor of pituitary, treatment with ACTH.

Clinical Features

See **Figure 7.6.**

CASE 7.5 DIABETES MELLITUS

History: Mr Sharma, 47-year-old obese man, attends your OPD with a complaint of tingling sensation in fingers. He has observed that he has an increased frequency of micturition and he feels thirsty all the time. Of late, he has an urge to eat more and more. The family history of type 2 DM present in the father and maternal grandfather. He has been on antihypertensive medication since 4 years.

Physical examination: The patient is calm, conscious, well oriented to time, place and person. He is overweight, weighing 85 kg and height of 170 cm. His vitals were recorded as temperature 98.6°F, pulse 78/min, regular and good volume. BP = 130/80 mm Hg. Systemic examination reveals no abnormality in abdomen, respiratory system and cardiovascular system.

Laboratory Investigations

Hb = 12 g/dL
Fasting blood glucose (FBS) = 240 mg/dL (normal: <100 mg/dL)
HbA1C = 8.5% (normal: 4–6%)

Lipid Profile

- Total cholesterol = 215 mg/dL (normal: <200 mg/dL)
- LDL cholesterol = 135 mg/dL (normal: <100 mg/dL)
- HDL cholesterol = 53 mg/dL (normal: >60 mg/dL)
- Triglycerides = 130 mg/dL (normal: <150 mg/dL)
- HDL: LDL ratio = 1.59:1 (normal: 2:1)

Renal Function Tests

- S. creatinine - 0.9 mg/dL (normal: 0.6-1.2 mg/dL)
- Blood urea nitrogen: 23 mg/dL (normal: 20–40 mg/dL)

Provisional diagnosis: Diabetes mellitus type-2.
- The syndrome caused by the deficiency of Insulin is called as diabetes mellitus.

Based on the above clinical scenario answer the following questions:
1. What is your probable diagnosis?
2. Explain the physiological basis for:
   a. Increase in frequency of micturition
   b. Increase in thirst
   c. Increase in urge to eat more
   d. Tingling sensation in fingers
   e. Increase in HbA_1C level.

- Criteria for diagnosing DM:
  1. Fasting blood glucose level: >= 126 mg/dL on 2 separate occasions
  2. Postprandial glucose level: >= 200 mg/dL at 2 hours

Classification

Primary DM

- **Autoimmune (Type IDM)**
  - Insulin dependent DM (Type I IDDM)
  - Non-insulin dependent DM (Type I NIDDM)
- **Non-autoimmune (Type II DM)**
  - Insulin dependent DM (Type II IDDM)
  - Non-insulin dependent DM (Type II NIDDM)

Secondary DM

- Due to any other cause
- Pituitary diabetes (due to persistent hyperglycemia)

Cause/Etiology

- **Autoimmune:** Antibodies to beta cells (Type I IDDM)
- **Genetic:** As seen in Type II NIDDM; due to HLA DR4
- **Infections:** Certain viral infections like measles and mumps results in damage to beta cells
- Persistant hyperglycemia due to other causes (secondary)
- Increase growth hormone level leads to increase of insulin → exhaustion of beta cells → failure of beta cells to produce insulin → DM
- Inflammation of pancreas

Clinical Features

Chief Complaints

- Excessive thirst, increased frequency of micturition, increased hunger (polydipsia, polyuria and polyphagia)
- Weight loss
- Increased susceptibility to infections
- Delayed wound healing

On Examination/Investigations

- Hyperglycemia
- Glucosuria
- Increased glycosylated Hb (HbA_1C)
- Ketosis
- Acidosis
- Hyperkalemia

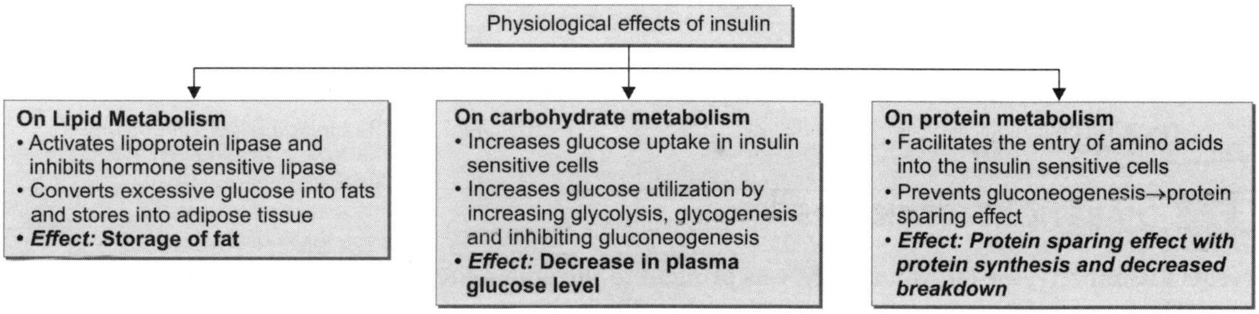

Fig. 7.7: Physiological actions of insulin on metabolism.

Table 7.1: Metabolic effects of deficiency of insulin.

Fat metabolism	*Carbohydrate metabolism*	*Protein metabolism*
Excess glucose is not converted into fat and stored fat is mobilized from adipose tissue into blood stream	Decreased glucose uptake by insulin sensitive cells and liver	Decreased uptake of amino acid in muscle
Inhibits lipoproteinlipase, which splits triglycerides in the blood into free fatty acids, which are stored in adipose tissue → Increases free fatty acids (FFA) in blood	**Increases plasma glucose level** (hyperglycemia)	Decreased synthesis of new protein
Stimulates hormone sensitive lipase, which splits stored TGs into FFA and releases into blood → Increases FFA in blood	Decreased utilization of glucose by *glycolysis*	Increased protein breakdown
	Decreased conversion of extra glucose into glycogen by *glycogenesis*	Increased uptake of AA by liver, *results in gluconeogenesis*
	Increased synthesis of glucose from fat and amino acids *(stimulation of gluconeogenesis)*	

Summary

Increases FFA in blood → promotes atherosclerosis and formation of ketone bodies (acetoacetic acid and β-OH butyric acid) → Acidosis	Increases plasma glucose levels (hyperglycemia) and decreases stores in the form of glycogen and fat because of in capability of cells to use glucose	Protein breakdown to produce glucose → increased plasma glucose levels (hyperglycemia)

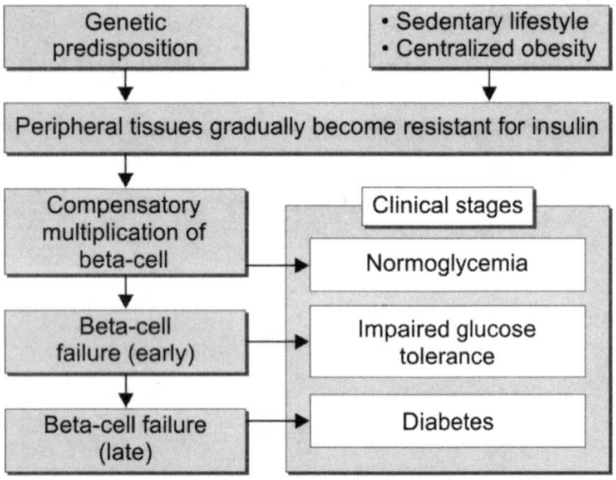

Fig. 7.8: Pathophysiology of diabetes mellitus type-2.

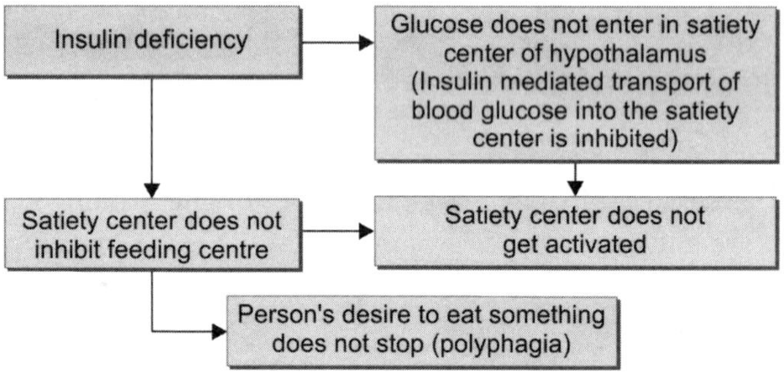

Fig. 7.9: Physiological basis of polyphagia.

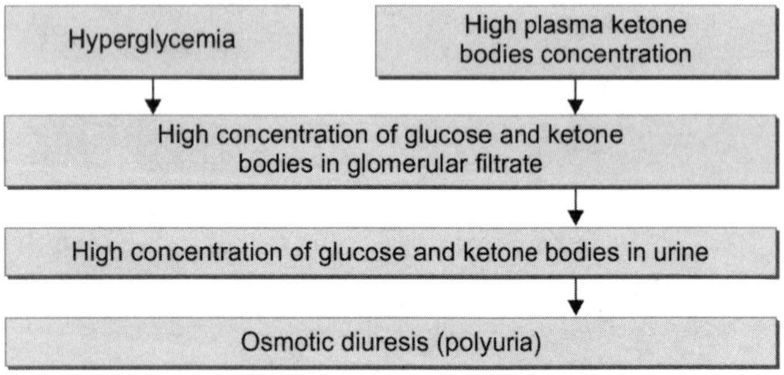

Fig. 7.10: Physiological basis of polyuria.

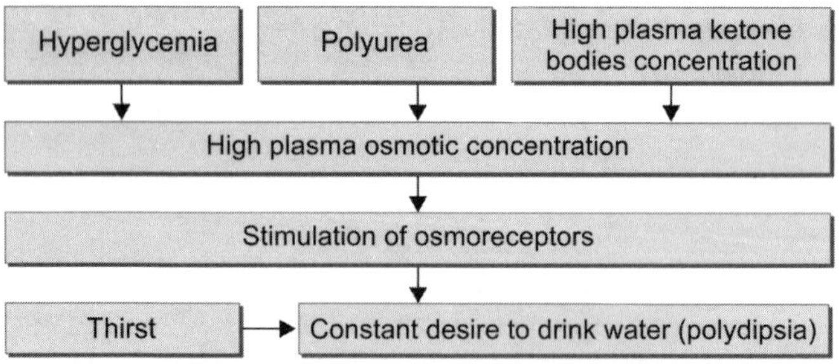

Fig. 7.11: Physiological basis of polydipsia.

CASE 7.6 DIABETIC KETOACIDOSIS

History: Ms Kusum, 27-year-old young lady, was brought to the emergency in a comatose stage with deep and rapid breathing. The mouth of the patient was dry and her breath was giving out fruity odor. She is a known case of juvenile diabetes since 18 years.

Physical examination: The patient was comatose and not oriented to time, place and person. She responded to the painful stimuli. She was lean and thin, weighing 48 kg and height of 160 cm. Her vitals were recorded as temperature 97.6°F, pulse 118/min, regular and low volume. BP = 100/60 mm Hg. Systemic examination revealed a tender abdomen. She had Kussmaul's respiration with ketotic breath.

Laboratory Investigations

- Hb = 10 g/dL
- Fasting blood glucose (FBS) = 520 mg/dL (normal: <100 mg/dL)
- HbA1C = 9% (normal: 4–6%)
- Na^+ = 138 mEq/L (normal: 135-145 mEq/L)
- K^+ = 4.6 mEq/L (normal: 3.5-5.5 mEq/L)
- Arterial pH = 7.0 (normal: 7.40)
- HCO_3^- =12 mEq/L (Normal: 23–30 mEq/L)
- Anion gap (Na^+ - (Cl^- + HCO_3^-): 15 mEq/L (Normal: 12 mEq/L)
- Plasma ketone bodies: ++++ (Normal: Absent)
- Urine glucose: ++++ (Normal: Absent)
- Urinary ketones: Present

Based on the above clinical scenario answer the following questions:
1. What is your probable diagnosis?
2. What is the pathophysiology of this disease?
3. Explain the physiological basis for:
   a. Increased level of plasma ketone bodies
   b. Glucosuria
   c. Low body mass index
   d. Increased anion gap

Provisional diagnosis: Diabetes mellitus type-1 diabetic ketoacidosis.
Definition: It occurs due to lack of insulin and excess of glucagon. Most common in Type II DDM. If production of ketone bodies is more than its destruction, there occurs ketosis or ketonemia. It occurs due to lack of insulin and excess of glucagon and most common in Type I IDDM.

Pathophysiology of Diabetic Ketoacidosis

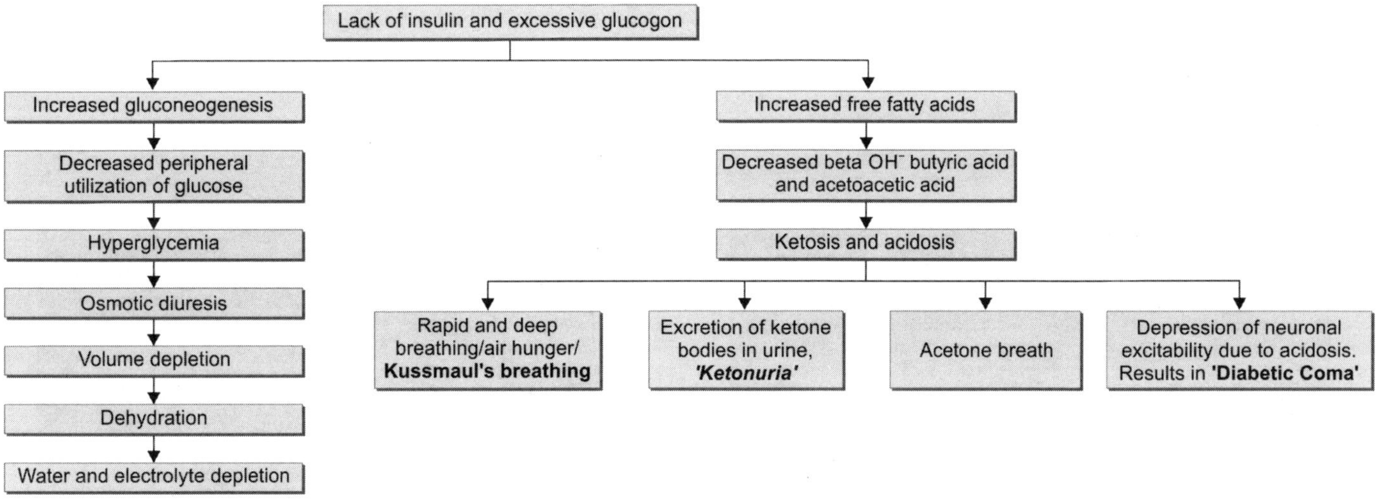

Fig. 7.12: Clinical features of diabetic ketoacidosis.

Signs and Symptoms

- Anorexia
- Nausea and vomiting
- Polyuria
- Abdominal pain
- If not treated → altered sensorium and coma

- Signs of dehydration
- Rapid and deep breathing → Kussmaul breathing
- Acetone breath

Lab Findings

- Very high blood glucose levels (475–750 mg/dL)
- Low sodium
- High potassium
- Raised BUN
- Ketone bodies ++
- FFA raised

Physiology of Management

- **Infusion of insulin:** It increases the uptake of glucose and potassium by the insulin sensitive cells, decreasing the blood glucose and serum potassium levels.
- **Fluid replacement:** It is done to correct the dehydration caused due to hyperglycemia, osmotic diuresis and hemoconcentration.
- **Potassium replacement:** It is done once the S. potassium levels drop due to increased uptake of potassium inside the insulin sensitive cells.
- **Bicarbonate therapy:** To correct the acidosis.

CASE 7.7 PRIMARY HYPERPARATHYROIDISM

History: A 40-year-old male patient complained of frequent constipation and loss of appetite. He had a previous history of renal stones.

Clinical Examination

- Temperature—normal
- Radial pulse—76 pulse/minute
- Blood pressure—110/70 mm Hg

Lab Investigations

- Plasma calcium level—13 mg/dL (normal range—8.6–10 mg/dL)
- Plasma phosphate level—decrease
- PTH level—230 pg/mL (normal range—15–65 pg/mL)
- Plasma vitamin D level—normal
- X-ray investigation

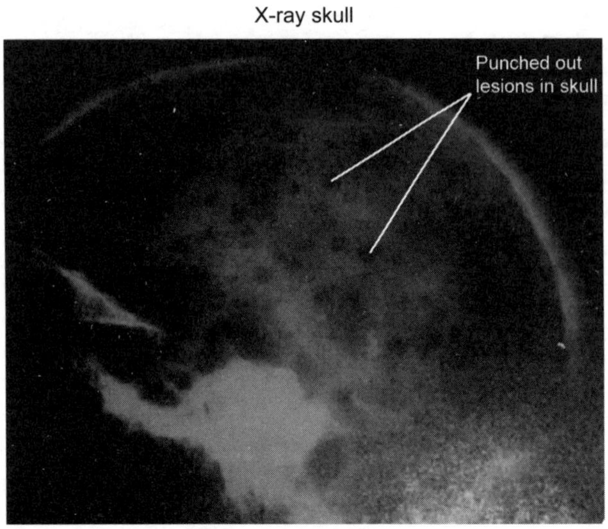

Fig. 7.13: Skull X-ray report showing salt and pepper sign.

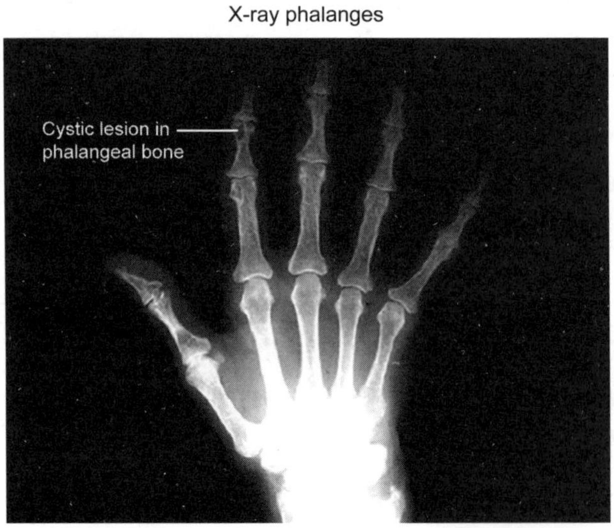

Fig. 7.14: Hand X-ray report showing subperiosteal bone resorption of phalanges.

Based on the above clinical scenario answer the following questions:
1. What is your probable diagnosis?
2. What is the pathophysiology of this disease?
3. Explain the physiological basis for:
    a. Renal stones
    b. Constipation
    c. Bone resorption (visible in X-ray findings)
4. What is brown tumor?

Diagnosis: Primary hyperparathyroidism.

At first look, the clinical features do not seem to highlight any specific direction for the diagnosis. So let's have a look at the investigation findings.
- Elevated PTH level and normal level of vitamin D
- Elevated plasma calcium level but decreased plasma phosphate level
- X ray findings are indicating toward bone resorption

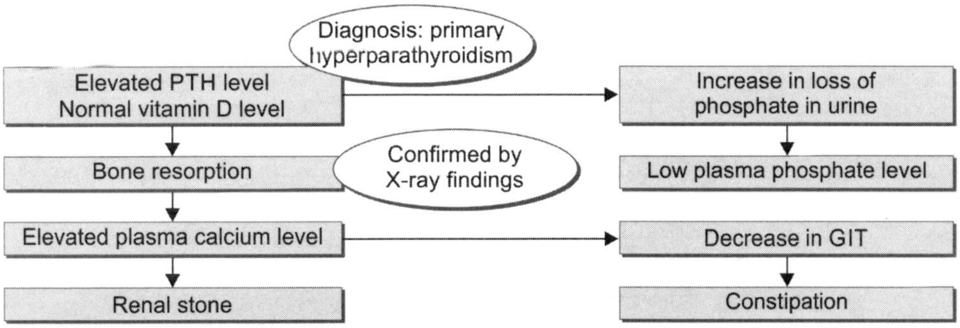

Fig. 7.15: Physiological basis of clinical features of primary hyperparathyroidism.

In some chronic cases we also see one more manifestation of bone resorption—"Brown tumor."

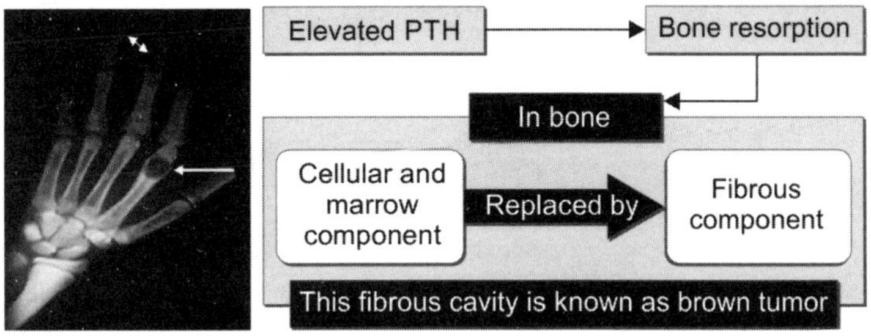

Fig. 7.16: Physiological basis of brown tumor in hyperparathyroidism.

The above described case scenario depicts primary hyperparathyroidism. However, if there is raised parathyroid levels in a patient of chronic renal failure resulting in bone reorption and all the above findings, it hints towards the secondary hyperparathyroidism.

CASE 7.8 SECONDARY HYPOPARATHYROIDISM

History: A 40-year-old male underwent complete thyroidectomy (removal of thyroid gland) due to previously diagnosed hyperfunctioning thyroid nodule. During the postoperative period, he complained of circumoral numbness and tingling.

On Examination

- Temperature—normal
- Pulse rate—76 pulse/minute
- Blood pressure—110/70 mm Hg

Tapping over the facial nerve resulted in twitching on that side of the face (positive Chvostek sign). Raising the pressure in the BP cuff, tied over the arm of the patient, precipitated muscular spasm in the hand (positive Trousseau's sign).

Lab Investigations

- Plasma calcium level—7.6 mg/dL (normal range—8.6–10 mg/dL)
- PTH level—05 pg/mL (normal range—15–65 pg/mL)
- Plasma vitamin D level—normal

Based on the above clinical scenario answer the following questions:
1. What is your probable diagnosis?
2. What is the pathophysiology of this disease?
3. Explain the physiological basis for:
   a. Positive Chvostek's sign and Trousseau's sign?
   b. Increased neuromuscular hyperexcitability?

Probable diagnosis: Post thyroidectomy hypoparathyroidism.

After the removal of the parathyroid gland during thyroidectomy, the serum calcium levels fall below the normal range resulting in hypocalcemia. All the clinical features of hypoparathyroidism, in this case, are due to hypocalcemia.

Pathogenesis

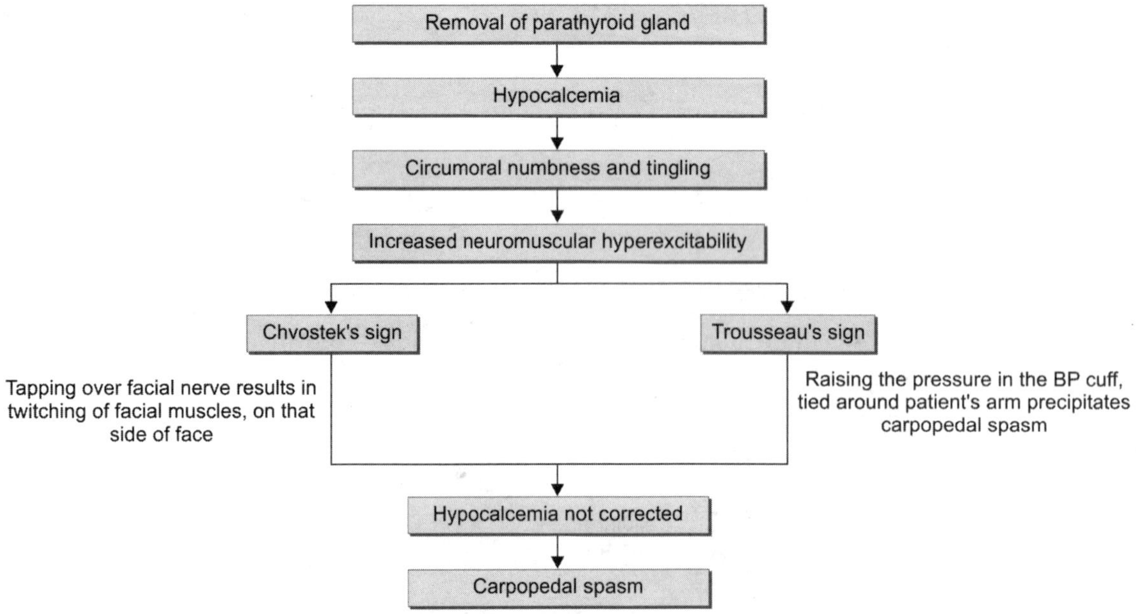

Fig. 7.17: Physiological basis of carpopedal spasm in post-thyroidectomy hypothyroidism.

The increased neuromuscular hyperexcitability, in a patient of hypocalcemia can be explained by the **Figure 7.18.**

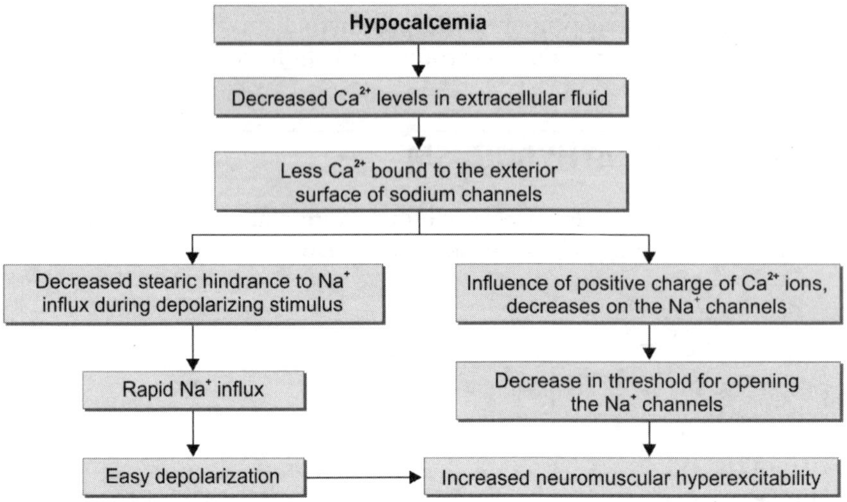

Fig. 7.18: Physiological basis of hypocalcemia induced increased neuromuscular excitability.

CHAPTER 8

Reproductive Physiology

PY9.8: Describe and discuss the physiology of pregnancy, parturition and lactation and outline the psychology and psychiatry-disorders associated with it.
PY9.9: Interpret a normal semen analysis report including (a) sperm count, (b) sperm morphology and (c) sperm motility, as per WHO guidelines and discuss the results.
PY9.12. Discuss the common causes of infertility in a couple and role of IVF in managing a case of infertility.
PY9.10 Discuss the physiological basis of various pregnancy tests.

LEARNING OBJECTIVES

After finishing this module, you should be able to:

- Analyze the clinical problem on the basis of its signs and symptoms, laboratory findings, to reach a differential diagnosis for that problem.
- Describe the pathophysiology of the given clinical condition based on the clinical and laboratory findings.
- Discuss the rationale of management, based on the derangement of physiological parameters in a case scenario.

CASE 8.1 MALE INFERTILITY

A 30-year-old male with a married life of 5 years, farmer by occupation was investigated as a case of primary infertility. He does not have any history of loss of libido, erectile dysfunction or history suggestive of any other systemic illness.

Past history: No history of tuberculosis or mumps.
Personal history: Occasional smoker and alcohol drinker.

On Examination

- No pallor/icterus/cyanosis/clubbing/pedal edema/generalized lymphadenopathy
- Secondary sexual characters normal
- Vitals: PR—82/min, BP—130/90 mm Hg
- Systemic examination—normal
- Examination of the scrotum and testes—normal

Lab Investigations

- **CBC:** Normal
- **Hormone assay:** Normal
- **Semen analysis:** Volume—2 mL, liquefaction time—completed after 30 minutes
- **Sperm count:** 8 million/cmm, motility—40% sperms are motile, sperm morphology—normal, pus cells, epithelial cells and RBCs are absent.

Based on the above clinical scenario answer the following questions:

1. What is the cause of infertility in this patient?
2. What is the normal semen analysis report?

Provisional diagnosis: Male infertility.

Table 8.1: Normal semen analysis (WHO guidelines 2010 updated in 2020).

Parameter	*Normal value*
Sperm volume (mL)	1.5
Sperm concentration (10^6/mL)	15
Total sperm number (10^6/ejaculate)	39
Progressive motility (PR,%)	32
Total motility (PR + NP + %)	40
Vitality (live sperms, %)	58
Sperm morphology (NF, %)	4
pH	≥ 7.2
Leukocyte (10^6/mL)	<1

CASE 8.2 NORMAL PREGNANCY

A young female with a married life of 6 months approaches a gynecologist with complaints of one and a half months amenorrhea.

Patient has a normal menstrual cycle of 28 days.

She has no history of similar complaints in the past and is not using any contraceptive method. She believes that she could be pregnant and wants to confirm the same. There is no other significant past medical or surgical illness.

Based on the above clinical scenario answer the following questions:
1. Which test can be used for detecting pregnancy?
2. What is the physiological basis of the pregnancy test ?
3. What are the physiological changes in a mother during pregnancy?

Provisional diagnosis: Normal pregnancy.

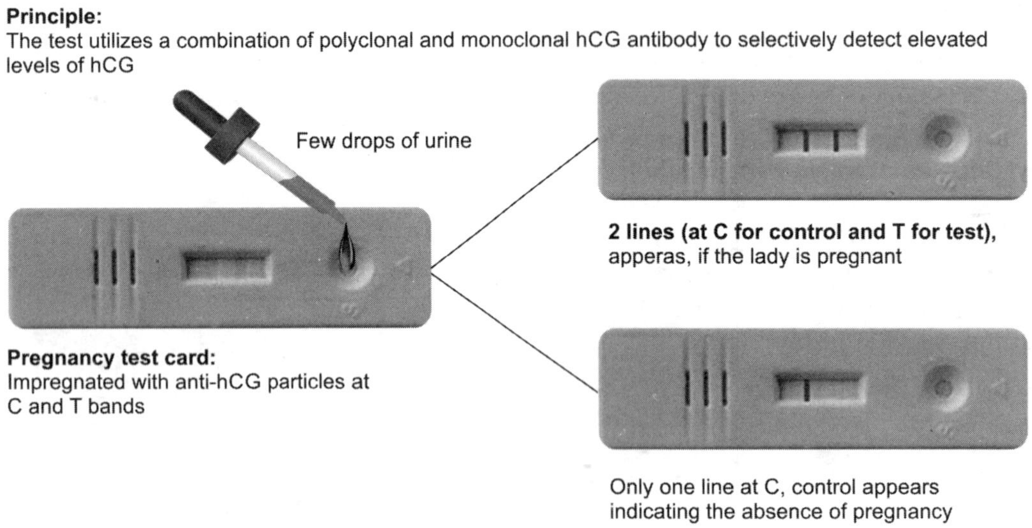

Fig. 8.1: Physiological basis for immunological test for pregnancy. Note: HCG begins to appear in the urine 7–10 days after conception.

Physiological Changes During Pregnancy

- **Changes in blood:**
  - Increased plasma volume (due to expansion of ECF volume; Na^+ and H_2O retention)
  - Increased red cell mass (due to increased erythropoietin)
  - Relative hemodilution (Increased PV/Decreased RBC count)
  - Physiological anemia of pregnancy
  - Moderate leukocytosis
  - Increased procoagulant activity due to increased synthesis of coagulation factors by estrogen

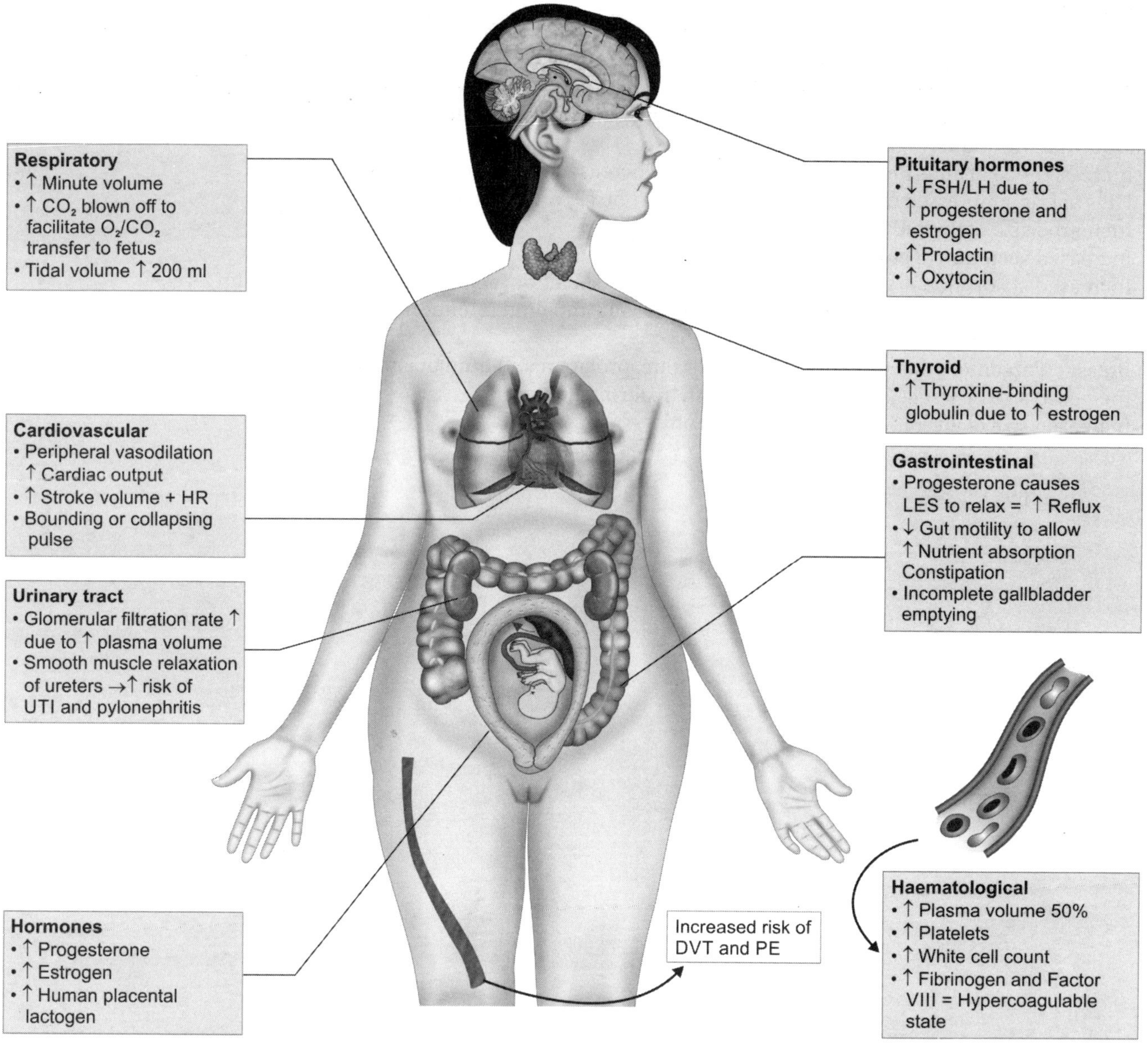

Fig. 8.2: Physiological changes during pregnancy.

(FSH: follicle stimulating hormone; LH: luteinizing hormone; LES: lower esophageal sphincter; DVT: deep vein thrombosis; PE: pulmonary embolism; UTI: urinary tract infection; HR: heart rate)

- **CVS:**
  - Increased CO, SV, HR, SBP
  - Decreased DBP due to vasodilation under the effect of progesterone
- **Respiratory system:**
  - Stimulation of respiratory centers by estrogen
  - Increased tidal volume (TV), inspiratory reserve volume (IRV), inspiratory capacity (IC) and minute ventilation
  - Decreased residual volume (RV), functional residual capacity (FRC) and expiratory reserve volume (ERV)
- **Kidneys:**
  - Increased renal blood flow and glomerular filtration rate (GFR)
  - Glycosuria
- **GIT:**
  - Decreased GI motility
  - Constipation
  - Reflex esophagitis towards term

- **Hepatobiliary system:**
  - Decreased serum proteins (dilutional hypoalbuminemia)
  - Increased serum alkaline phosphatase
  - Increased plasma lipid and cholesterol (due to inhibition of lipoprotein lipase)
  - Decreased bile flow (inhibition of CCK induced gallbladder contraction by progesterone)
- **Endocrinal functions:**
  - Increased size of anterior lobe of pituitary due to increased prolactin secreting cells
  - HPO axis is suppressed due to increased progesterone (P) and estrogen (E)
  - Increased size of thyroid gland; iodine deficiency
  - Increased secretion of glucocorticoids and mineralocorticoids
  - Increased absorption of Ca^{2+} from gut; increased PTH secretion → increased plasma calcium levels
- **Body weight gain:** Due to fat deposition by progesterone and fluid retention
- **Breasts:**
  - Breast enlargement due to estrogen, progesterone, prolactin and human chorionic somatomammotropin (HCS)
  - Increased size of areola and nipple along with hyperpigmentation
  - Increased size of alveoli → alveolar hypertrophy.

9 CHAPTER Neurophysiology

PY 10.6 Describe and discuss spinal cord, its functions, lesion and sensory disturbances.
PY 10.7 Describe and discuss functions of cerebral cortex, basal ganglia, thalamus, hypothalamus, cerebellum and limbic system and their abnormalities.
PY 10.9 Describe and discuss the physiological basis of memory, learning and speech.

LEARNING OBJECTIVES

After finishing this module, you should be able to:

- Analyze the clinical problem on the basis of its signs and symptoms, laboratory findings, to reach a differential diagnosis for that problem.
- Describe the pathophysiology of the given clinical condition based on the clinical and laboratory findings.
- Discuss the rationale of management, based on the derangement of physiological parameters in a case scenario.

CASE 9.1 BROWN-SEQUARD SYNDROME

History: After falling from the stairs, a 62-year-old man complained of loss of touch sensation in the left lower limb and stiffness in the right lower limb.

On examination: His vitals were normal with temperature 98.6°F, pulse 76/min, BP = 136/76 mm Hg. He was conscious, calm and well oriented to time, place and person.

Examination of CNS Revealed

- Loss of all sensations in the right side of the body 1 cm above umbilicus and flaccid paralysis.
- Loss of fine touch, proprioception, two point discrimination and vibration in right side of body below the area of complete anesthesia along with spastic paralysis, exaggerated deep reflexes and lost superficial reflexes in right side of body.
- Loss of touch, temperature, pain and pressure sensation in the left side of body, 2 cm below the area of complete anesthesia, with no motor abnormality.

Based on the above clinical scenario answer the following question:

1. What is your probable diagnosis?
2. What is the pathophysiology of the disease?
3. How will you determine the level of lesion?
4. Why there is flaccid paralysis at the level of umbilicus?
5. What is the cause of spastic paralysis below the level of lesion?
6. Which tracts are involved in carrying the sensations and how are they involved in this injury?

Provisional diagnosis: Hemisection of spinal cord (Brown-Sequard syndrome).

An injury to the spinal cord, in which half of the spinal cord is transected, is called Brown-Sequard syndrome.

Level of lesion: As seen in the figure, there is complete loss of sensation and flaccid paralysis, 1 cm above the umbilicus, hence the level of lesion is 1 cm above umbilicus (T10 dermatome), i.e., T9 level, on the right side. But because of tract of Lissauer, the actual injury is 1–2 segments below the clinical presentation of injury. Hence, the actual site of injury in this patient will be at T10/T11.

Motor Loss

- There is lower motor neuron type of lesion at T9 dermatome due to damage of lower motor neurons (alpha motor neurons)
- There is upper motor neuron type of lesion below T9 dermatome due to loss of inhibition of stretch reflex arc by the higher/upper motor neurons resulting in hyperactive stretch reflex and spastic paralysis, below the lesion on right (ipsilateral) side.
- There is no motor loss seen in the contralateral side of lesion.

Sensory Loss

- There is loss of all the sensations at T9 dermatome.
- Due to damage to dorsal column tract, the sensation of fine, touch, tactile discrimination, tactile localization, proprioception, vibration are lost.
- Due to damage to anterior and lateral spinothalamic tracts, the sensation of crude touch, pressure, pain and temperature are lost.

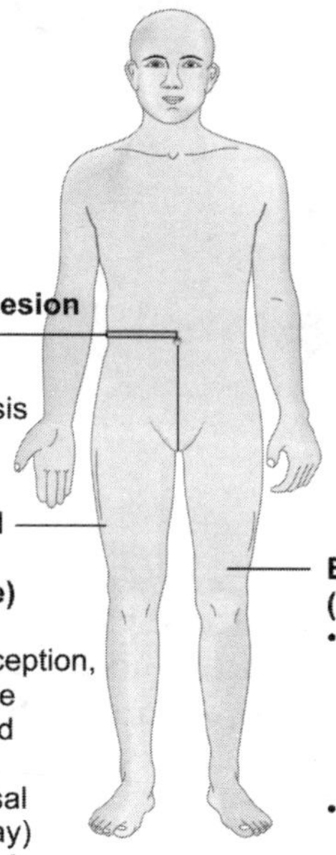

Fig. 9.1: Clinical features of Brown-Séquard syndrome.

CASE 9.2 PARKINSON DISEASE

History: Harish, a-60-year-old male, reported difficulty in initiating any motor activity like walking, brushing his teeth, etc. He also mentioned that, with aging, his motor activities had become slower. Doctor also noted that while he was sitting, there were tremors in his hand. On further questioning, Harish mentioned that these tremors stop while doing any activity. Doctor also noted that, along with the change in emotions, there was no change in facial expressions.

On Examination

His vitals were normal with temperature 98.6°F, pulse 75/min, BP = 130/80 mm Hg. He was conscious, calm and well oriented to time, place and person.

The general facial expressions of the patient were lost resulting in a mask-like face.

Examination of CNS Revealed

- **Motor functions:**
  - *Tone:* Hypertonia with cogwheel type rigidity in limbs.
  - Power of muscles is Grade +4/+5.
  - *Reflexes:* Deep tendon reflexes are normal. Plantar response is flexor.
  - Pill rolling resting tremor of the hands.
  - Shuffling gait with narrow base and a tendency to fall forward and backwards. He walks with slight flexion at hip and knee joints.
  - Cerebellar function tests are normal.
- **Sensory function:** Normal.
- **Cortical sensations:** Normal.
- **Higher functions:** Normal.

Based on the above clinical scenario answer the following question:

1. What is your probable diagnosis?
2. What is the pathophysiology of the disease?
3. What is the physiological basis of hypokinetic (akinesia, bradykinesia) clinical feature?
4. What is the physiological basis of hyperkinetic (tremors, rigidity) clinical features?

Provisional diagnosis: Parkinson disease.

First of all, let's jot down some of the peculiar symptoms and clinical findings which would lead us to the final diagnosis:

- Elderly person
- Difficulty in initiating movement (akinesia)
- Slow execution of motor activity (bradykinesia)
- Tremors in resting state (resting tremors)
- Hypertonia
- Shuffling gait

All these symptoms and clinical findings are pointing towards "Parkinson disease", as the probable diagnosis.

Pathophysiology of Parkinson Disease

Basal ganglia is consist of 4 nuclei:

1. Striatum (caudate nuclei + putamen) (STN)
2. Globus pallidus [intrena (GP_{IN}) and externa (GP_{EX})]
3. Subthalamic nucleus (STN)
4. Substantia nigra [divided in—pars compacta (SNPC) and pars reticulata (SNPR)]

These structures are interlinked by direct and indirect pathways.

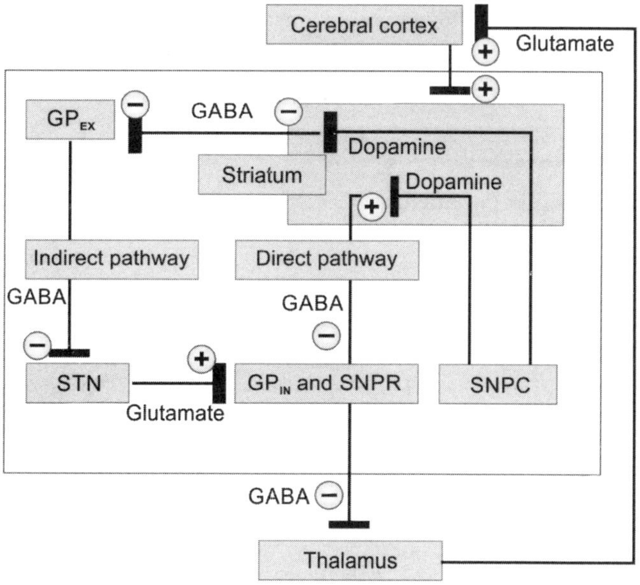

Fig. 9.2: Direct and indirect circuits in basal ganglia.

As the **Figure 9.2** shows, dopamine has stimulatory effect on direct pathway and inhibitory effect on indirect pathway. Direct and indirect pathway influence the final basal ganglia output through GP_{IN} and SNPR. Parkinson disease involves degeneration of substantia nigra. It leads to decrease in dopamine secretion through nigrostriatal pathway. Because of this decrease in dopamine secretion, the tone of inhibitory basal ganglia output increases. In this way, through thalamus, basal ganglia increases the inhibitory effect on motor cortex and it manifest as hypotonia, akinesia, bradykinesia and loss of associated movements.

Now the next question is—what is the cause of hyperkinetic features, like—resting termers, and rigidity? We would like to refer to a hypothesis proposed by scientists. According to this hypothesis, these hyperkinetic features might be because of pacemaker-like activity of some thalamic nuclei which gets unmasked due to increased inhibitory output from basal ganglia.

CASE 9.3 CEREBELLAR ATAXIA

History: A 30-year-old male non-smoker, social drinker was admitted as a case of motor vehicle accident. On admission patient was diagnosed to have suffered from severe concussion and fracture left radius. Patient was hemodynamically stable. Surgical repair of the fractured left radius was done. Neurological assessment of the patient show that patient had poor balance and postural instability.

On Examination

- During the hospital stay
- Vitals stable
- CNS examination: Patient conscious, well oriented to time, place and person
- Saccadic eye movements present
- Other visual tests: Normal
- Sensory system examination: Normal
- Deep tendon reflexes: Normal
- Plantar reflex: Normal
- Cerebellar function test:
  - Intentional tremors present
  - In-coordinated movement of the right hand
  - Unable to maintain balance and standing posture.

Investigations

MRI: Right cerebellar hemisphere lesion.

Based on the above clinical scenario answer the following questions:
1. What is your probable diagnosis?
2. Explain the physiological basis for:
   a. Intentional tremor
   b. In-coordination in motor activity

Provisional diagnosis: Post-traumatic cerebellar ataxia.

Pathophysiology

Cerebellum also known as the little brain is a large collection of nuclei that control and coordinate motor activity. Functionally the cerebellum can be divided into 3 portions:
1. **Spinocerebellum:** Is this central portion.
2. **Cerebrocerebellum:** Is the lateral portion.
3. **Vestibulocerebellum:** Is the lower portion.

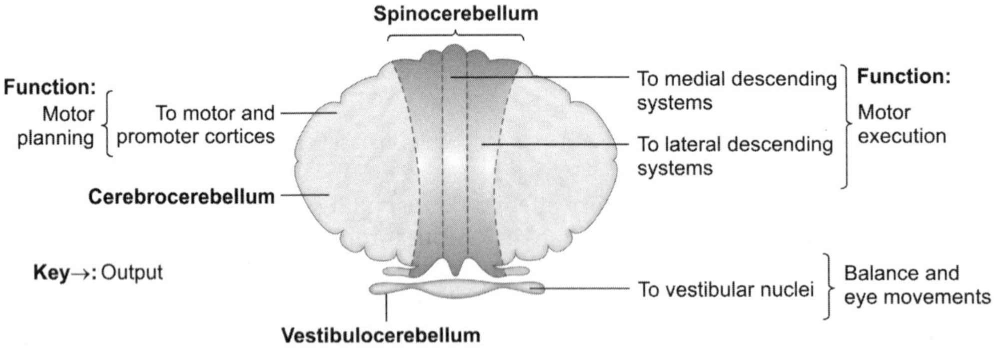

Fig. 9.3: Functional division of cerebellum.

A patient of cerebellar lesion presents with ataxia, intention tremor and uncoordinated movements.
- The patients with the lesions of the vermis, often present with truncal ataxia.
- Lesions of vestibular cerebellum result in in loss of equilibrium and balance in the posture maintenance.
- The occurrence of the intention tremor could be explained on the basis of the functional unit of the cerebellum, which result in the damping of the movement which is initiated by the climbing as well as mossy fibers. In case of cerebellar lesion, the movement initiated by these fibers is not damped, resulting in past pointing/overshoot and hence the intention tremor.
- It is this past pointing which hampers the repetitive movements, resulting in the uncoordinated movements in the cerebellar lesion.
- It is important to understand that a patient with cerebellar lesion will not be able to maintain his balance, perform the coordinated activity either with eyes open or closed, however a patient suffering from sensory ataxia will be able to perform the task with his eyes open but not when eyes are closed.
  Therefore the Romberg sign is positive with eyes open as well as eyes closed in patients of cerebellar dysfunction.

CASE 9.4 HEAT STROKE

History: A 28-year-old male was admitted to the emergency department by the relatives with complaints of nausea, vomiting, malaise followed by dizziness. The relative gives a history of trekking a day before the onset of symptoms. No other significant medical or surgical history in the past.

On Examination

- Patient is conscious, co-operative, mildly disoriented
- Temperature: 40°C
- Pulse: 98/min
- BP: 100/70
- RR: 18/min
- Skin: Red with hot, dry feel
- CVS examination: Normal except tachycardia
- Respiratory system examination: Normal except tachypnea
- CNS: Mildly disoriented and agitated

Based on the above clinical scenario answer the following questions:
1. What is your probable diagnosis?
2. What is the pathophysiology of the disease?
3. What are the basic mechanisms of regulating body heat?

Provisional diagnosis: Heat stroke.

Human body temperature is strictly maintained around 36.5°C +/-0.5°C by the central thermostat situated in the hypothalamus which sense change in the temperature inside the body and the peripheral thermoreceptors present on the skin which can sense change in the temperature outside the body. This strict temperature maintenance is crucial as all the metabolic processes in the body are temperature dependent.

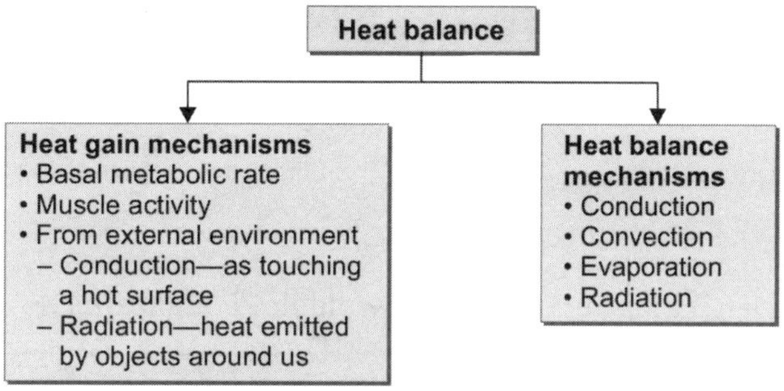

Fig. 9.4: Methods of heat balance.

Thermoregulation and heat balance is achieved by the body's specific homeostatic responses towards a hot and cold environment as shown in the table below:

Table 9.1: Temperature regulation during hot and cold weather.

Mechanisms	*Hot weather*	*Cold weather*
Heat gain		
1. Basal metabolic rate	Decreases	Increases by shivering
	Lethargy	Active
2. Muscle activity	Having cold food and beverages	Having hot food and beverages
3. Behavioral responses	Putting on fans, air conditioners	Putting off fans, air coolers
	Light clothing, etc.	Woollen clothing, etc.
Heat loss		
1. Conduction 2. Convection	Increased by vasodilatation	Decreased by vasoconstriction
3. Evaporation 4. Radiation	Increased sweating	Increased hyperventilation

In a hot environment the body tries to lose heat and in a cold environment the body tries to conserve heat.

CASE 9.5 APHASIA

History: A 70-year-old male presented with chief complaints of sudden onset of repetitive speech, restlessness and irrelevant talk.

- **Patient was apparently normal 2 hours back when he suddenly started repeating words which had no meaning and was not able to understand what the family was speaking.**
- **No history of fall or trauma, headache, nausea, vomiting, loss of consciousness, fever or any signs of weakness in the limbs.**
- **Patient is a known case of hypertension on regular treatment for last 10 years.**
- **No other significant medical or surgical illness in the past.**

On clinical examination
- No pallor/cyanosis/clubbing/edema or lymphadenopathy
- Vitals: Pulse: 78/min, BP: 190/100 mm of Hg, Temperature: Normal

CNS examination
Patient is conscious, irritable and agitated.

Speech
- Repetitive talks, neologism present
- Comprehension impaired
- Naming impaired
- Reading and writing: Non-cooperative

Motor examination: Normal.

Cranial nerve examination: Normal.

Cerebellar function test: Normal.

Investigations

- CBC: Normal
- LFT: Normal
- Renal profile: Normal
- Blood sugar: Normal
- S.electrolytes: Normal
- ECG: Within normal limits (WNL)
- Echocardiography: Normal
- CT brain normal
- CT angiography: Thrombosis of left parietal branches of the middle cerebral artery

Based on the above clinical scenario answer the following questions:
1. What is your probable diagnosis?
2. Damage to which area is responsible for the given clinical condition?
3. How will you differentiate between Broca's aphasia and Wernicke's aphasia?
4. Enumerate the speech areas in the brain.

Provisional diagnosis: Sensory aphasia.

Pathophysiology

Speech is defined as the ability to express oneself by spoken or written words and aphasia is speech disorder resulting from lesions in the brain.

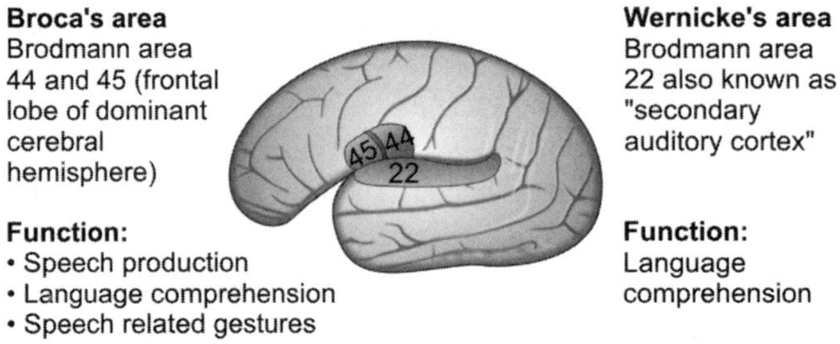

Fig. 9.5: Cortical areas associated with speech.

Table 9.2: Different types of aphasias.

Sensory aphasia/fluent aphasia	*Motor aphasia/non-fluent aphasia*	*Global aphasia*
Lesion: Damage to parts of the temporal lobe around Wernicke's area with intact Broca's area	**Lesion:** Is in the Broca's area with intact Wernicke's area	**Lesion:** Is in the perisylvian cortex including Wernicke's and Broca's area
Clinical features: • Defect in comprehension • Speech is nonsensical but fluent	**Clinical features:** • Defect in verbal/speech expression • Non-fluent • Effortful and slow	**Clinical features:** • Preserved comprehension • Fluent • Impaired repetition
Logorrhoea—irrelevant speech • Neologism • Jargon speech • Paraphasia	**Dysarthria** • Agrammatic speech • Poor word output • Poor pronunciation	

CASE 9.6 ALZHEIMER'S DISEASE

History: A 50-year-old male non-diabetic, non- hypertensive is brought to the family physician by her son with presenting C/o forgetfulness since last year, and since the last 2 months he has become more forgetful. Once-easy-tasks are becoming increasingly difficult such as placing a telephone call, following directions, and routine daily activities. He has difficulty naming objects and telling time.

- **He often does not recognize old friends and forgets previous conversations.**
- **No other significant medical or surgical history in the past**
- **Non-smoker, non-alcoholic with no known history of any drug abuse.**

On Examination

- Patient is not well oriented to time, place and person
- Averagely built and well-nourished
- Vitals: Normal
- Systemic examination: NAD

CNS

- Patient is not well oriented to time, place and person
- Mini-mental state examination (MMSE) test for cognitive function
- Score—20

Investigations

- Relevant blood investigations—normal
- MRI—show shrinkage in the frontal and temporal lobes
- Ct-scan—normal

Based on the above clinical scenario answer the following questions:

1. What is your probable diagnosis?
2. Differentiate between explicit and implicit memory?

Provisional diagnosis: Alzheimer's disease.

Pathophysiology

Alzheimer's disease is a common cause of dementia.

It is a chronic progressive neurodegenerative disease of the cerebral cortex with an insidious onset that gradually affects the cognitive functions finally causing deficits of memory (short-term memory), physio-spatial orientation, judgment, language and personality.

Patients suffers from:

- Confusion, disorientation and getting lost in familiar places
- Has a problem with activities of daily living

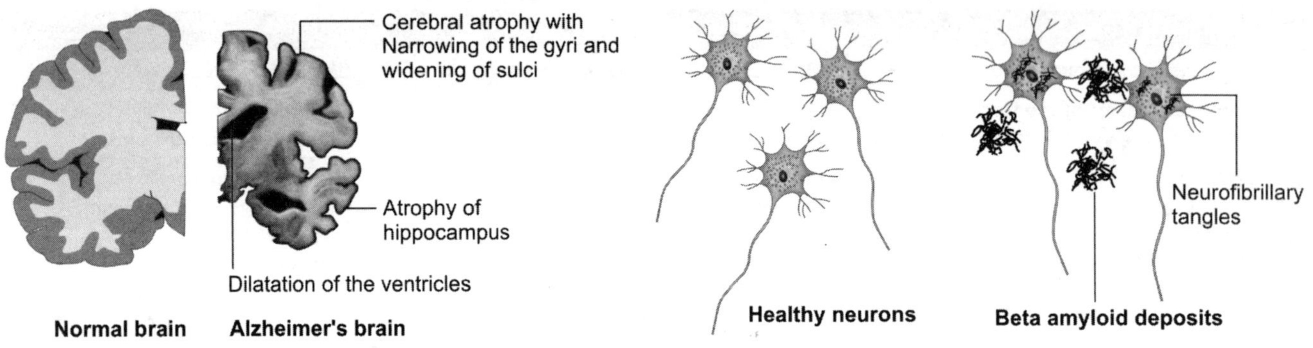

Fig. 9.6: Cortical and neural changes in Alzheimer's brain.

- Speech and language problems
- Planning or making decisions becomes difficult
- Personality changes
- Hallucinations and delusions
- Low mood or anxiety

Alzheimer's disease is characterized by the deposition of two types of abnormal proteins in the brain particularly the *hippocampus* which is responsible for learning and memory especially explicit memory and the *prefrontal cortex* which governs the cognitive abilities, i.e., the daily routine activities, thought process, decision making ability.

Beta amyloid plaques which cluster outside the neurons and the Tau proteins inside the neurons which form neurofibrillary tangles.

These beta amyloid plaques cause:

- Inflammatory responses
- Prevent synaptic transmission and disrupt neuronal metabolism (glutamate reuptake mechanism)
- Risk of intracranial hemorrhage by getting deposited in the blood vessels.

10 CHAPTER Physiology of Special Senses

PY 10.17 Describe and discuss functional anatomy of eye, physiology of image formation, physiology of vision including color vision, refractive errors, color blindness, physiology of pupil and light reflex.
PY 10.18 Describe and discuss the physiological basis of lesion in visual pathway.

LEARNING OBJECTIVES

After finishing this module, you should be able to:
- Analyze the clinical problem on the basis of its signs and symptoms, laboratory findings, to reach a differential diagnosis for that problem.
- Describe the pathophysiology of the given clinical condition based on the clinical and laboratory findings.
- Discuss the rationale of management, based on the derangement of physiological parameters in a case scenario.

CASE 10.1 CONDUCTIVE HEARING LOSS

Nitesh, a 10-year-old boy, presented with complaints of pain in left ear with some degree of hearing loss. Since the last 4 days, he has been suffering from a sore throat.

On Examination

- Pulse—80/min
- Body temperature—99.5 F
- Lymph node examination—enlarged left cervical lymph nodes
- Examination of both ears:

Table 10.1: Tuning fork test for hearing.

Examination	*Finding*	
	Left ear	*Right ear*
Rinne's test	AC < BC	AC > BC
Weber test	**Lateralized to left ear**	
Schwabach test	Patient's BC was better than the examiner's BC	Patient and examiner had equal BC
ABC test	Patient and examiner had equal BC	Patient and examiner had equal BC

(AC: air conduction; BC: bone conduction)

Based on the above case, answer the following questions:
1. What is your provisional diagnosis?
2. What does a positive Rinne's test indicate?
3. Why Weber's test is lateralized to left ear?

Provisional diagnosis: Conductive hearing loss.

Pathophysiology

Patient seems to be suffering from conductive hearing loss in the left ear. It might be because of acute otitis media (acute middle ear infection) because of primary upper respiratory tract infection. For better understanding of this diagnosis let's take a look at the findings of clinical findings with the possible explanations.

- Mild fever and lymphadenopathy could be due to acute infection.
- Cochlear nerve examination.
- The Weber's test is lateralized to the deaf ear in case of conductive deafness, because of masking and the presence of ambient environmental noises in the healthy ear. However, it is lateralized to the healthy ear in sensory neural deafness due to the damage to the hair cells, resulting in the loss of the auditory signal.

Table 10.2: Differentiating feature of normal ear and deaf ear on the basis of tuning fork tests.

Hearing test	*Normal hearing*	*Conductive deafness*	*Nerve deafness*
Rinne's test	Positive (AC>BC)	Negative (AC<BC)	Positive (AC>BC) Though AC is less than normal
Weber test	Equally heard in both ears	Lateralized to deaf ear	Lateralized to normal ear
Schwabach test	Equal in subject and examiner	Subject's BC is better than the examiner's BC	Examiner's BC is better than the subject's BC
ABC test	Equal in subject and examiner	Equal in subject and examiner	Examiner's BC is better than the subject's BC

CASE 10.2 PRESBYCUSIS

A 80-year-old male had a complaint of difficulty in hearing in both ears. On further questioning he mentioned that it was a gradual hearing loss. No significant medical and surgical history in the past.

On Examination

- Vitals: Normal
- Systemic examination: No significant abnormality detected
- Examination of both ears:

Table 10.3: Tuning fork test.

Examination	*Finding*	
	Left ear	*Right ear*
Rinne's test	AC > BC	AC > BC
Weber test	**Equal in both ear**	
Schwabach test	Examiner's BC was better than the patient's BC	Examiner's BC was better than the patient's BC
ABC test	Examiner's BC was better than the patient's BC	Examiner's BC was better than the patient's BC

(AC: air conduction; BC: bone conduction)

Pure tone audiometry: Decrease in sensitivity for all the sound frequencies.

Based on the above case, answer the following questions:
1. What is your provisional diagnosis?
2. What is cause of this condition?

Provisional diagnosis: Presbycusis.

Definition: Presbycusis is age—related hearing loss characterized by gradual hearing loss affecting both the ears symmetrically.

Type: Sensorineural deafness affecting higher pitched sounds more than low pitched sounds.

Pathophysiology

Causes: Loss of hair cells, neurons in the cochlea and atrophy of stria vascularis that regulates the endolymph.

- It is seen more in males
- Incidence increase with increase in the age

- Loud noise exposure during lifetime
- Hearing examination.

Management

- Hearing aids to amplify sounds
- Cochlear implants

CASE 10.3 MYOPIA

A 13-year-old girl has complaints of frequent headaches and difficulty in seeing far objects clearly. It was affecting her school studies as she was unable to see things written on the blackboard clearly. She did not face any difficulty in reading a book or observing near objects.

On Examination

- Visual acuity for far vision (using Snellen's chart): 6/9 for left eye, 6/9 right eye (Normal: 6/6)
- Visual acuity for near vision (using Jaeger's chart): N_8 in both eyes
- Field of vision (using confrontation test): Normal in both eyes
- Color vision (using Ishihara's color plates): Normal
- Pupillary reflexes: Normal reaction to light and accommodation in both eyes

Based on the above case, answer the following questions:
1. What is your provisional diagnosis?
2. Enumerate the various refractive errors.
3. Which lens is used for correction of myopia and why?

Provisional diagnosis: Myopia.

Definition: Myopia or nearsightedness is a refractive error in which the parallel rays of light coming from a distant object are focused in front of the retina so the patient is not able to see distant objects clearly.

Pathophysiology

- Increase in the curvature of the lens or cornea
- Increase in the axial length of the eye increases the converging power
- Increase in the refractive index of the lens, e.g., in cataract
- Anterior displacement of the lens as in case of trauma

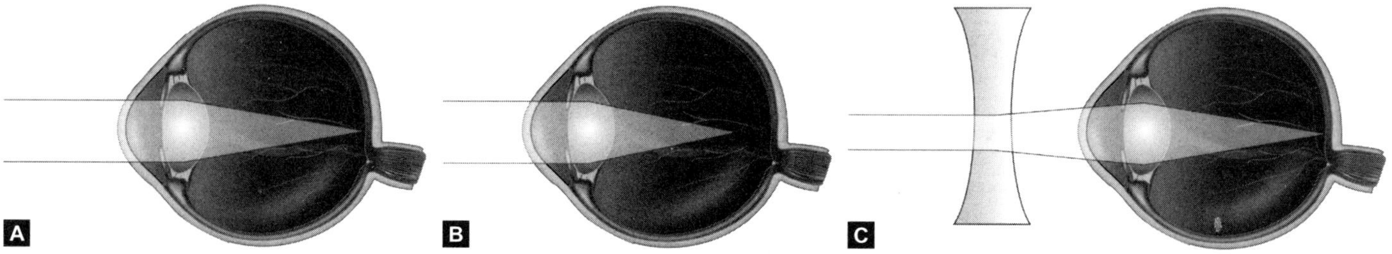

Figs. 10.1A to C: (A) Normal eye: Parallel rays of light from a distant object are focused on the retina ; (B) Myopic eye: Parallel rays of light from a distant object are focused in front of the retina ; (C) Correction of refractive error: Use of concave lens.

CASE 10.4 PRESBYOPIA

A 50-year-old female had difficulty in visualizing near objects since few years and now this problem has become big enough to affect her day to day work. There is no trouble seeing distant objects.

On Examination

- Visual acuity for far vision (using Snellen's chart): 6/9 in left eye and 6/18 in right eye
- Visual acuity for near vision (using Jaeger's chart): N10 in both eyes

- Field of vision (using confrontation test): Normal in both eyes
- Color vision (using Ishihara's color plates): Normal
- Pupillary reflexes: Normal

Based on the above case, answer the following questions:

1. What is your provisional diagnosis?
2. What is the physiological basis of clinical features?
3. Which lens is used for correction of presbyopia and why?
4. What happens to far point and near point in presbyopia?

Provisional diagnosis: Presbyopia.

Definition: It is an age-related physiological process in which there is progressive worsening of the ability of the eye to focus on near objects usually seen after the age of 40 years.

Pathophysiology

After the age of 40 years the near point (punctum proximum) recedes beyond the normal range. Hence the power of accommodation decreases with age resulting in loss of power of accommodation. Due to loss of accommodation in presbyopia, the far point becomes nearer and near point becomes far. Hence bifocal convex lenses are used for correction of presbyopia.

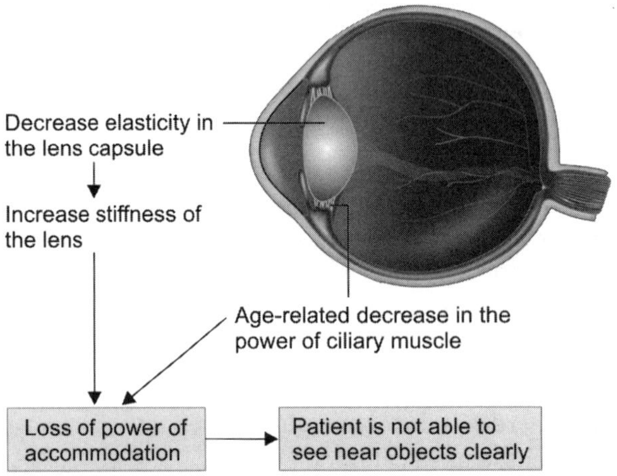

Fig 10.2: Pathophysiology of presbyopia.

CASE 10.5 DEFECTS IN VISUAL PATHWAY

A 35-year-old male patient who is a known case of acromegaly comes to the ophthalmologist with complaints of obscured side vision.

On Examination

- **GPE:** Prominent supra-orbital ridges, thick lips, exaggerated nasolabial, protrusion of the jaw, large hands and feet.
- **Vitals:** Normal.
- **Visual acuity for near and distant vision:** Normal.
- **Confrontation test:** Patient could not see the finger from the temporal side of both the eye.

Investigations

- **CT scan:** Pituitary adenoma.
- **MRI:** Pituitary adenoma compressing the optic chiasma.

Based on the above case, answer the following questions:
1. What is your provisional diagnosis?
2. Draw a well labeled diagram showing the various visual field defects.

Provisional diagnosis: *Bitemporal hemianopia due to underlying pituitary adenoma.*

This patient who is a known case of acromegaly due to pituitary adenoma, which is compressing the optic chiasma, results in the compression of the optic fibers present within it.

The diagram of the visual pathway with various visual defects, due to the lesions arising are shown below:

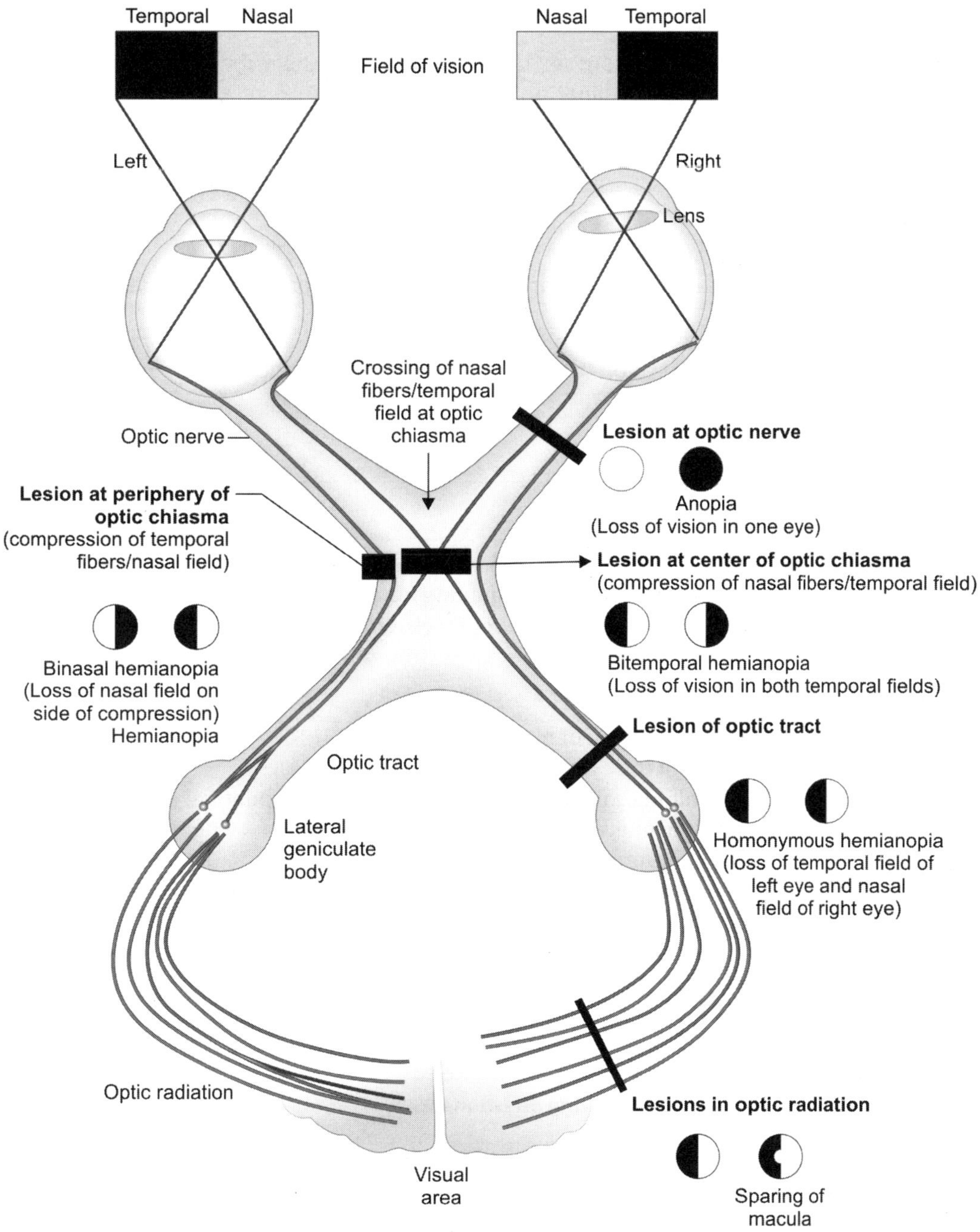

Fig. 10.3: Effects of lesions at various levels of visual pathways.

11 CHAPTER Physiology of Chromosomal Aberrations

PY 9.1 Describe and discuss sex determination; sex differentiation and their abnormalities and outline psychiatry and practical implication of sex determination.

LEARNING OBJECTIVES

After finishing this module, you should be able to:
- Analyze the clinical problem on the basis of its signs and symptoms, laboratory findings, to reach a differential diagnosis for that problem.
- Describe the pathophysiology of the given clinical condition based on the clinical and laboratory findings.
- Discuss the rationale of management, based on the derangement of physiological parameters in a case scenario.

CASE 11.1 DOWN'S SYNDROME

History: A 16-year-old male patient, fourth birth order, born to a non-consanguineous couple was referred to the Department of Orthodontics with the chief complaints of spacing between teeth in the upper as well as the lower jaws. The patient also complained of missing teeth and desired replacement of the same.

On Examination

- The patient is moderately built with a mild degree of mental retardation.
- Short palpebral fissures, epicanthic folds of the eyelid causing almond shaped.
- Eyes, brushfield spots on the iris, mongoloid slant, depressed nasal bridge, and bilateral clinodactyly.
- The patient also has a short neck, and abnormally shaped ears, small hands and feet, deep crease in the palm of the hand, single palmar fold, i.e., Simian crease, poor muscle tone.
- Intraoral examination revealed generalized spacing of teeth in relation to the maxillary and mandibular arches and the clinical crowns were conical and smaller than normal (microdontia). The patient had a high arched palate, relatively small mouth and macroglossia with a crenated tongue. He also presented a descending angle of the mouth, and an everted lower lip with tongue protrusion.
- Family history was non-significant.
- Medical history was unremarkable except for delayed milestones of development.

Based on the above clinical scenario answer the following questions:
1. What is your probable diagnosis?
2. What are the other clinical conditions that can present with mental retardation?

Provisional diagnosis: Down's syndrome.
Definition: Down's syndrome also called as Trisomy 21 or mongolism. Chromosomal abnormality arising due to nondisjunction of chromosome 21.

The child is born with an extra copy of chromosome no 21 resulting in gene excess abnormalities.

Pathophysiology

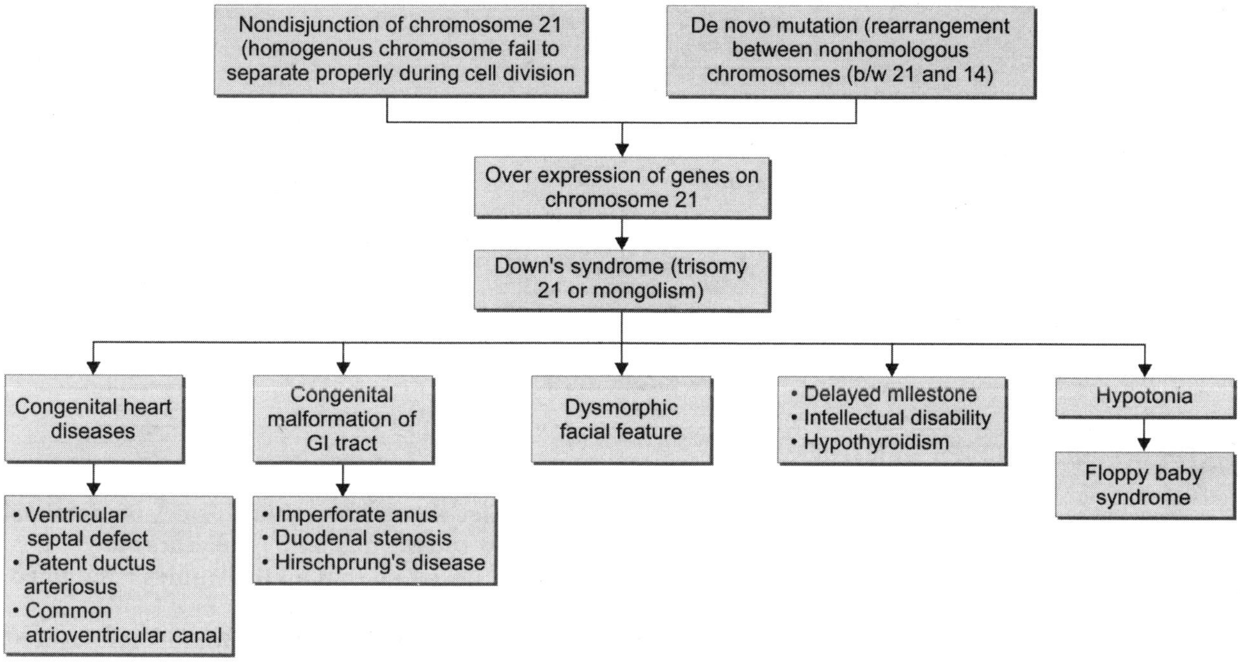

Fig. 11.1: Pathophysiology of Down's syndrome.

CASE 11.2 TURNER'S SYNDROME

History: A 16-year-old girl was brought to the endocrinologist referred by a gynecologist with features of short stature, webbed neck and primary amenorrhea.

She is the second child born by Cesarean section to non-consanguineous parents the age of mother was 28-year at the time of her birth. Milestones of development Normal, no history of any genetic disorder or mental retardation in the family. Her elder sister had normal menarche.

On Examination

- Height: 133 cm
- Lack of axillary and pubic hair with underdeveloped breast [Tanner stage-I]
- Broad chest and widely spaced nipples
- External genitalia appear to be normal

Investigations

- USG—small sized uterus with absent ovaries
- Hormone assay—high follicular stimulating hormone (FSH) levels

Based on the above clinical scenario answer the following questions:
1. What is your probable diagnosis and enumerate the important features to support your diagnosis?
2. What is the karyotype of this female?
3. What are the anomalies can you expect in this patient?

Provisional diagnosis: Turner's syndrome.

Definition: Turner syndrome is the most common sex chromosomal abnormality in phenotypic males and results due to the loss or abnormality of the second X chromosome. Karyotype of Turner syndrome is 45 XO in 80% of the cases.

Characteristic features Include:
Short stature webbed neck, broad chest with widely spaced nipples, primary amenorrhea with primary infertility and other cardiac and renal anomalies.

Pathophysiology

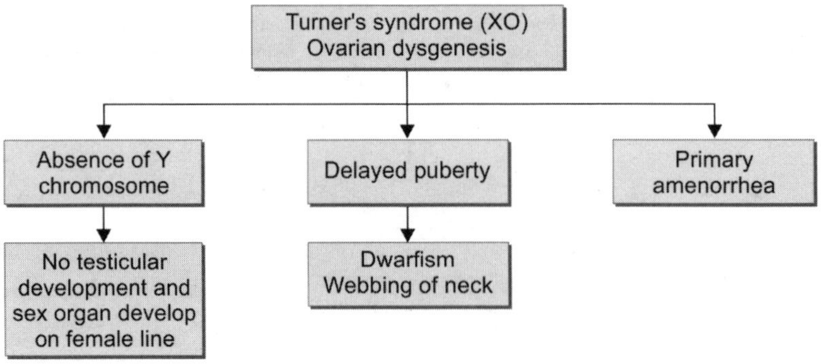

Fig. 11.2: Pathophysiology of Turner's syndrome.

CASE 11.3 KLINEFELTER'S SYNDROME

History: A married couple comes to the endocrinologist referred by a fertility center with a history of married life of 3 years and trying to conceive for the last 2 years. The wife is 26 years old and the husband is 28 years old.

After taking a proper history and reviewing the previous reports it observed that all the studies conducted on her were normal and the female factor as a cause of infertility was hence ruled out.

Husband's semen analysis showed Azoospermia and was referred to the endocrinologist for further evaluation.

On Examination of the Husband

- **General physical examination:** No pallor/cyanosis/clubbing/edema/lymphadenopathy. Patient is tall with scanty and sparse facial and body hair distribution, reduced muscle mass. Gynecomastia and small testes.
- **Vitals:** Temp-N, BP: 120/80 mm of Hg, Pulse: 86/min.
- Examination of the respiratory system cardiovascular system and central nervous system showed no significant abnormality.

Based on the above clinical scenario answer the following questions:
1. What is the probable diagnosis of infertility in this couple?
2. What other test will you suggest for the male partner to support your diagnosis?

Provisional diagnosis: Klinefelter's syndrome.

Definition: Klinefelter syndrome is a chromosomal disorder due to the presence of an extra copy of X chromosome, i.e., 47 XXY. The individual is genetically female with the genitalia of a normal male.

Pathophysiology

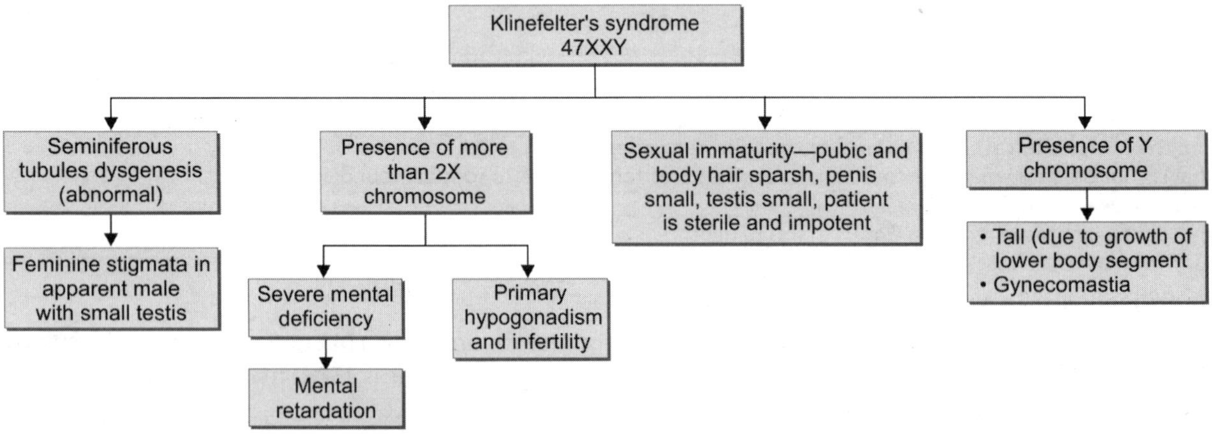

Fig. 11.3: Pathophysiology of Klinefelter's syndrome.